MY MISSION STATEMENT

'To connect women to the moon cycles and the
seasons. Releasing stress and overwhelm, to restore
balance, motivation, gain clarity, direction, and align
to your goddess power. Readying you to sparkle and
shine, dancing through your life and spreading your
unique medicine and magic.'

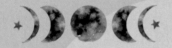

2024

Moon Goddess diary

NORTHERN
HEMISPHERE

THIS DIARY BELONGS TO THIS GORGEOUS BEING:

_____

ROCKPOOL

Beloved,

This year I have called in, united and gathered from across the world, 12 of the most powerful goddesses who have worked with my energy across the dimensions of time.

Each goddess is unique, radiant and has her own individual medicine to weave through the pages of this diary.

Each one has her own way to connect to the sacred feminine energy that resides within you.

Each goddess is choosing to be there to teach and guide you this year. They are there for you now.

Imagine my surface. See 12 goddesses there: standing, dancing, mixing potions, singing, playing music, making magic, swimming in my waters and looking over the earth where you are now.

Use their knowledge. Feel their power. Bathe in their love. Breathe in their radiance.

Just as you do so with me.

Loving you through each moment,

Grandmother Moon xx

PS: Should you ever feel the need for that extra support, big beaming sign of love or reminder that you are incredibly important and so worthy of being seen, you only need to look up. I'm always here.

ABOUT THE AUTHOR

Hey!

I'm Nicci, a moon dancer, ocean soul, goddess, mother, lover, pleasure seeker and creator of fun who is dedicated to helping you become the woman you most want to be.

I am a transformational speaker, kinesiologist, medical intuitive and energy healer who is incredibly connected to the angelic realm, the beautiful mother earth wisdom and to all those shamanic guides and practices.

My four children, Summer-Rose, Harmony, Trinity and Maverick are the focus of my world and not a day goes by that I am not wowed by the love and support they all give to me.

I'm an Aussie girl who tries to breathe fun and pleasure into my every day. I love to feel beautiful, sexy, fulfilled and supported. I have a dream that ALL women need to allow themselves to rise up. Embracing their divine feminine, their intuitive knowings and the connection to their soul, their goddess energy and living from this profoundly magical space.

I'm proud to have created this diary that inspires women all over the world to feel connected to the cycles of the moon and the seasons. To feel worthy and ready to live from their highest potential by 'tuning in' to their desires and prioritizing themselves and their pleasure.

Women are often raised and encouraged to fit into this world by being the caregivers, the nurturers, playing small, being a certain size, shelving their dreams for the sake of their family. So often we shelve our natural way of doing things, the way of feeling into something, our intuition and our fun for the benefit of others.

For me, this is where I found the moon and she guided me back to myself when I had become lonely and lost on my journey of trying to answer the question 'Who am I?' This was an awakening for me.

This diary encourages you to be you, all of who you are, and help you find the way back inside. I've done it and you can too!

I am so honored to have you join me for this year. It's going to be powerful, magical and completely awesome.

Nicci xx

INTRODUCTION

I started these diaries because full moons are the perfect opportunity and gift to each of us to release and clear away anything that you feel is no longer in your highest good. I used to go down to my local beach and sit under the full moon two to three times a year to balance my body, my cycles, my emotions and my systems. I'd meditate, walk in the sand, stand with the waves licking over my feet – a bit like hitting a reset button, just for me.

It was a wonderful reason to have a whole hour to myself without the kids too! My clients across the world were looking for similar things to help them hit their reset buttons so they could discover their sacred space or ceremony to come back to themselves.

In December 2016, I started my Full Moon Meditations offering my clients the opportunity to come down to the local beach where I lived in Queensland, Australia to meditate under a full moon. That first month we had 20 people come. We watched the moon rise and as I held the space for these women, we meditated together. Within three months we had over 100 people coming. Just outside of a year, we reached over 2,500 people filling the beach. In January 2019 we had over 4,500 people attend that night.

The moon really does affect us all. By choosing to harness this energy and by having the awareness found in this diary and accessing your goddess self-care toolkit, you will feel balanced, aligned and supported. You will begin thriving as you become the empowered woman you are truly destined to be.

I see you,

Nicci xx

> PS: The 2024 edition of this dairy was written in a little apartment above a coffee shop in Darlinghurst NSW, down the road from Sydney Harbour, the Oxford Street rainbow crossing and across the road from the Sydney School of Arts. It is infused with extra healing powers of diversity, of being who you are, of cosmopolitan vibes and abundant creativity medicine extracted from all around this beautiful place.

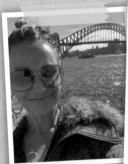 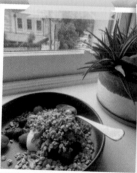 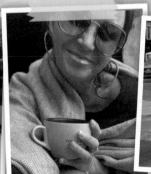 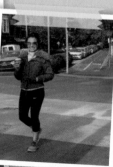

HOW TO USE THIS DIARY

This diary is written with the intention that you write, draw, color, paint, paste and doodle in it. Its pages are longing for you to fill them each week with sprinkles of your love. Sometimes when you get a new diary, a little part inside of you stirs up – it's a resistance to actually putting anything in your pages that may not be right, may not be good enough or could be judged. You may feel it's imperfect or it's something you feel ashamed about and you regret putting it in, and so on. It's all just your fears (usually from when you were at school) about being imperfect and not enough.

Let's do a quick ritual to bring healing to this area so that you are free to play, express and communicate throughout the course of your diary and also your year.

Hold your diary open (it doesn't matter which page) and start to breathe deeply, in and out. Settle into your body with your calming breath, slow it down and allow your breath to find a rhythm of its own … that's it.

Surround yourself, your diary and the whole space around you with a beautiful, soft pink light. This pink light completely surrounds you with an upgraded, safer and more potent way for you to express yourself through your diary. It activates your capacity to connect to those inner parts of your deep heart space yearnings and your intuitive self, so you can be more open to expressing yourself in ways that you love. This pink light is the color of your heart medicine and it will stay with you throughout your journey in 2024.

Scrawling, scribbling, gluing, messy, neat, organized, print, SHOUTING CAPITALS, curse words, drawing, stick figures, pictures, images, color, texta, crayons, kid's drawings, stickers, post-it notes, cut-outs, words, quotes, incorrect grammar, punctuation and spelling mistakes are all welcomed and allowed to be present within the pages of your diary. And so it is.

Call in the magic and the medicine of the 12 sacred goddesses who have been channeled in to support you this year with their guidance, their love and their radiance; call in Ishtar, Lemanja, Dewi Ratih, Yolkai Estsan, Devana, Aine, Coyolxauhqui, Lakshmi, Ch'ang-O, Hecate, Haliya and Mayari and weave in their magic even more throughout your whole body and the pages of your diary.

Take three deep breaths to come back into this moment, feeling excited to play in your diary and feel supported by your 12 goddesses from across the world throughout 2024. Gosh, it's going to be such an incredible year for you.

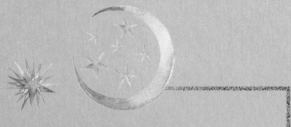

MY GODDESS SELF-CARE TOOLKIT FOR WINTER

All moon goddesses have tools that help them do their job better, easier, quicker or smarter, like secret weapons of support. Creating a few really specific, powerful and different self-care tools will help bring you the support you need to cope and thrive through each season of this year. These tools will help you show up to be the best version of yourself each day.

Life gets messy, drama happens, things don't always go as planned, you get emotional, the moon stirs the energy up and some days you can feel like 'it's all too much'. Having the tools to support you through these times is what propels you through them rather than falling in a heap of 'why bother' or 'I can't do this anymore'. These tools help you stay in the moment of your life and reconnect to your inner potency of awesomeness. They will help you find your magic and sparkle.

You outgrow things that support you because you are always changing and growing and shifting. You will find yourself choosing different tools to support you for each season. You will notice your personal shift and how your needs change with each season. And that's important.

Winter is the time of retreat, clearing and taking the time to get to know yourself deeper so you may be reborn in the spring, stronger and ready to bloom. All the self-care tools you choose here will support you from today until the spring equinox in March. These self-care tools will help you thrive throughout your winter season with an extra infusion of love and magic.

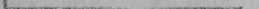

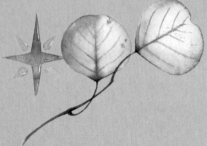

GODDESS MEDICINE

Let's start with choosing a goddess. Flip through until you come to January, February and March. Really notice the picture of each goddess and read the description about her. Which goddess feels like she will help you the most this season? The goddess I have chosen to support me throughout winter 2024 is:

_____

She will support me with the medicine of her

_____

COLOR MEDICINE

Choose one color that is going to support you throughout winter. Land on your color and write it down here:

_____

When I see this color, I feel

_____

I can use this color to support me throughout winter with things such as clothing, accessories, jewelry, flowers, scatter cushions, candles, crystals, pens and

_____

SOUND MEDICINE

Choose three songs. Songs that you love, songs that get you up and moving, songs that make you feel that it's impossible to stay completely still, songs that make you feel like you want to boom-shakka-lakka and shimmy-shake around your house. When you feel irritated, what could you do to get those deep irritations and emotions out of your body? You can dance them out! Yes, I know it sounds a little bit weird (okay, super weird) but it really does work. If I am feeling a little triggered, angry, scared, irritated or just in a funk, I can play these three songs so I can get all loose and not caring, and allow the music and dance to move me through the emotion.

My three songs are:

1. _____

2. _____

3. _____

Your song mission is to download your three songs and create a special winter playlist on your phone so that, whenever you need them, they are ready for you.

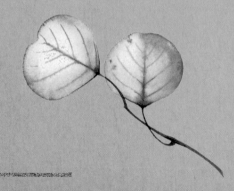

BODY MOVEMENT MEDICINE

Moving your body is important: you know that, I know that, everyone knows that. If there was a magical place that you could visit and it would transform your body with the push of a button, we'd all go there, right? Unfortunately, I am yet to discover this place so, for now, we all have to move our bodies to keep them strong, healthy and bendy in the ways we have available to us at this moment. Choose an exercise that feels as joyful, pleasurable, enlightening and as fun as it can be. There are so many ways to move your body. Choose one that feels exciting for you now.

The ways I will move my body during winter are:

_____

I will do these at _____ (location), _____ times per week.

PLANT MEDICINE

Botanicals have been used for thousands of years to support us to stay healthy and strong. Using different plants, their flowers or their fruit to cure ailments, support you to sleep better, help you to feel more vital, boost your immunity, encourage your digestive system to function easier, balance your hormones or help you feel more energized makes you feel like you are supporting your well-being.

Choose one health focus for winter. Write it here:

_____

Now research your focus and commit to taking or using this plant medicine each day throughout winter. You can find so many ways to bring in the magic of plants like supplements, teas, tinctures, essences, rubs or even a fresh bunch of herbs. Remember that tablets, teas and so on don't work if they stay in the cupboard, they need to be used!

AROMATHERAPY MEDICINE

Your nose is a powerful tool. When you smell something you love, your whole body feels so happy. It is like your nose holds this secret power to connect you to what brings you pleasure. You may even have memories triggered by your sense of smell. In choosing to notice these scents you love and by sprinkling them throughout your day, you will trigger a pleasure response that reminds you to feel all loved up and amazing. Kinda cool, hey! For winter, choose one smell that is going to support you throughout this season. It could be an essential oil, a perfume, a flower. Choose something you just love that is easy to use and fills you with pleasure.

Land on your fragrance and write it down here:

_____

When your nostrils are tickled with this fragrance, how do you feel?

_____

I can use this fragrance as my signature winter scent to support me in lots of ways such as burning essential oils and candles, using in skincare, eating or cooking with it, wearing the perfume, smelling fresh flowers, as well as

_____ and _____

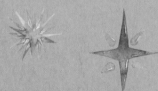

CRYSTAL MEDICINE

Crystals are like magical particles that hold healing powers within. There are thousands of crystals available and they all have individual characteristics or ways to support you. Using the magic of one crystal helps to guide you with what you are working on, with healing, clearing or reminding you how you are growing and what you are wanting to step into. The crystal I am choosing to support me for winter is called

_____

It is _____ (color) and it will help me to _____

I can use this crystal to support me in lots of ways, such as carrying a piece in my pocket, or keeping a piece in the car or my bag. I could wear it in jewelry, use it as a screensaver on my phone, pop it under my pillow or mattress to support me while I sleep, or I could

_____ or _____

For an extra gold star for being amazing, fill in three things you love most about winter.

1. _____

2. _____

3. _____

I will choose to do these things more because they bring me pleasure and fill my heart with joy. I deserve joy. (Yes, you really do!) Well done. That is your very own goddess self-care toolkit for winter all finished and completed. It will be here to support you through to the spring equinox in March. Call in your goddess and play your three songs now, swaying those hips as you dance and twirl around in celebration of completing your toolkit and being so special.

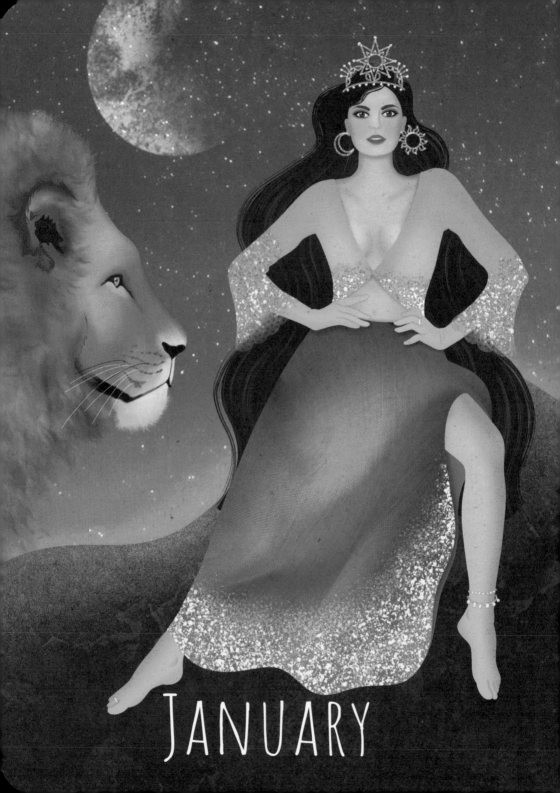

JANUARY

ISHTAR

Ishtar — whose earlier name was Inanna — was worshipped in the ancient lands of Babylonia, Mesopotamia, Akkadian, Assyria and Sumeria (now known as Iraq and parts of Syria and Turkey). She is the goddess of love, beauty, desire, sensuality, fertility, sex and war. She has a very strong connection to the planet Venus and is known as 'Queen of the Night' and 'Daughter of the Moon' making her your powerhouse Moon Goddess for this month.

As the goddess of love, Ishtar is an incredible example of walking to the beat of your own drum and infusing your life with love, pleasure, dancing, play and choosing your desires. She weaves in through this month the magic of being fun and flirty, feeling beautiful and sexy, and the importance of filling your life with things, animals, experiences and people you love.

Ishtar is teasing out of you the radiant, divinely feminine soul who is inside you, inviting you to really own your feminine vitality, power and fierceness.

Ishtar's mantra is 'I am learning that as I exquisitely love myself, life supports me to own my power.'

Her crystals are lapis lazuli for her connection to her deeply held wisdom and for being authentic.

Her totems are lions for power and the 8-pointed star associated with the planet Venus.

Her exercises are all things dance — tribal, Latino, belly, pole, hip-hop, ballet, and so on.

Her scents are alluring and sacred such as saffron, sandalwood, frankincense and rose.

I MONDAY

Sending you blessings and radiant love sprinkles for a very Happy New Year, beautiful one. Twirl around with your arms open wide and fully stretched out to the possibility of this year. 2024 is going to be amazing, powerful, filled with exquisite love, your best and most fabulous year yet. Feel into that expansion, that hope and pull it down into your heart space.

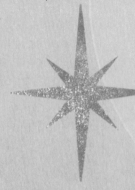

2 TUESDAY

3 WEDNESDAY

4 THURSDAY ◑

5 FRIDAY

2024 is a number 8 in numerology 2+0+2+4=8. The themes for number 8 years are personal power, success, abundance, pleasure and infinite possibilities. 2023 was a year where your focus was on connecting deeper to your wisdom so you could begin moving forward in your life, adding meaning to what you want and why you want it.

   In 2024 you have this incredible energy of feeling empowered, of holding your confidence and working with it in each moment. Of reaping the benefits of all your hard work and trusting that you're supported to choose your dreams and opening to receive it all.

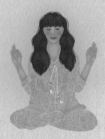

6 SATURDAY

7 SUNDAY

8 MONDAY

9 TUESDAY

10 WEDNESDAY

The dark nights of the waning moon are a time of such sacredness and magic. This lead up to the new moon birthing brings you this gift of beautiful, mystical nights that hold the space for you to let go of anything that you have been holding on to, allowing it to dissolve away.

It's like a surrendering to all that is going on in your life right now, a softening into acceptance and love. A pause. How can you pause today?

11 THURSDAY ○

Happy new moon, darling one. Today, new waves of magical moonbeams spread through your world offering you waves of love and light. The first new moon of 2024 falls in the earthy sign of Capricorn so stability, focused direction and grounded movement into your year is what's coming through.

Choose right now to live this year on purpose with arms wide open – ready to embrace your divine radiance and using this beautiful new moon energy to spark the excitement, the love, the magic and invite in your potency to be the sexy creator of your life.

Loving you ... to the moon and back.

12 FRIDAY

13 SATURDAY

14 SUNDAY

15 MONDAY

16 TUESDAY

Ishtar's message for you – 'Today I invite you to look at the ways you are different from those around you. Notice your differences. Lean into them. Feel them. Love them. It is in the getting to know yourself that you may just discover what makes you truly sacred and very special.'

17 WEDNESDAY

18 THURSDAY

Ishtar has a strong connection to the planet Venus: the planet of love, sensuality, pleasure and harmony. Imagine you are calling in a connection to this planet today, call down the magical channel of pink light and connect it into your heart space. Feel it filling up your body with exquisite love beams. How can you choose your pleasure, your sensuality today?

19 FRIDAY

20 SATURDAY

21 SUNDAY

22 MONDAY

The energetics of your first full moon for 2024 will start to brew this week. Remember that you have your goddess self-care toolkit to support you this year ... so use it, baby.

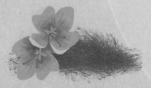

23 TUESDAY

24 WEDNESDAY

25 THURSDAY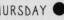

Happy full moon, sweetheart. Falling in the sign of Leo, this moon is stirring your desires and passions, deeply reawakening your fire and whispering to you to be brave and bold. It's time to discover what turns you on; to call in your creativity, to find your joy, your flirty playfulness, your fun and infuse these through your life.

This moon really paves the way for change. Feel into the possibility of what your life can look like when you are brave, when you can embrace new ways of doing things and when you can embrace your inner flirt – her sparkly glow.

26 FRIDAY

27 SATURDAY

Wear something bold and sexy this weekend, something that turns you on, date yourself, and love that precious one you are ... extra exquisitely.

28 SUNDAY

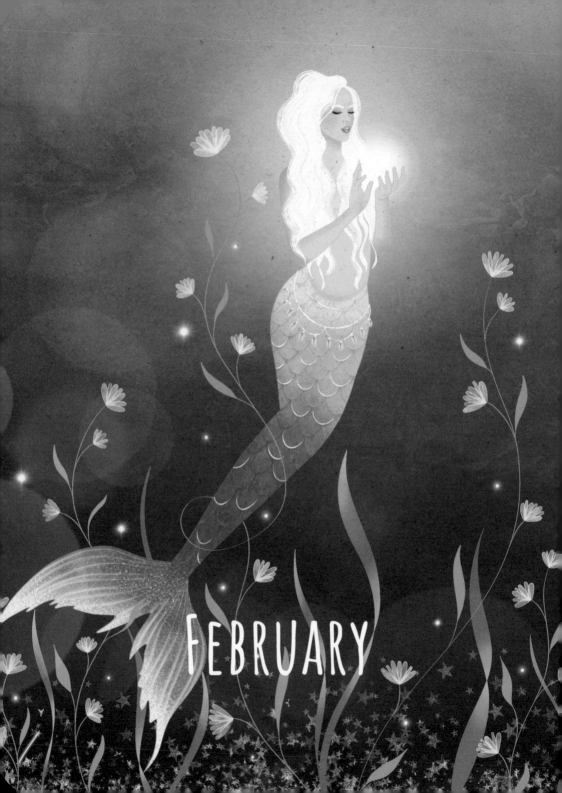

February

LEMANJA

Lemanja (Yemanja) is a beautiful goddess of the sea, of women and of the ocean and is often associated with the moon and its cycles. Lemanja is your moon goddess for February as across Brazil, Cuba, Uruguay and Africa she is lovingly worshipped and celebrated this month.

Ancient myths associate Lemanja with everything to do with the divine feminine; the cycles, fertility, mothering, birthing, creating life, sensuality and she fiercely protects everything around the mysteries of womanhood. It is said that when Lemanja's waters broke in childbirth and gushed from within her, this is how the sea, the oceans, the lakes and the streams were created. She birthed humans from her womb; she is the creator, giver and protector of life.

Lemanja is depicted here as a beautiful mermaid with cowrie shells, swimming in the depths of the ocean and holding the sparkle of moonlight within her hands that she sends to you to support you this month to birth your projects into reality.

Lemanja's mantra is 'I am learning that as I connect to my divine feminine my projects and creativity flow effortlessly from deep within me. I am the divine creator of my story.'

Her crystals are cowrie shells signifying her wealth and larimar for her connection to the sea.

Her totem is the white rose for purity and beauty.

Her exercises are all things in and on top of the water.

Her scents are peace and tranquility blends such as lavender, clary sage, cedarwood, lime and chamomile.

29 MONDAY

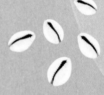

30 TUESDAY

31 WEDNESDAY

Ishtar's gift to you today is a sacred piece of lapis lazuli to place in your heart and carry with you for the rest of your year. She gives you this crystal so that you begin the journey of connecting to your deeply held wisdom and to remind you to be authentically you.

I THURSDAY

2 FRIDAY ◐

Lemanja asks you to notice how you feel and what's going on for you. You really are so very wise when you trust you have the answers you need. Look 'in' today and just notice how you feel. Trust in your inner knowings.

3 SATURDAY

4 SUNDAY

5 MONDAY

Remember that Lemanja is with you, deepening your connection to the sacred wisdom of the world and the nature spirits that are all dancing in your dreams today.

It's just a thing that everyone believes in you. (Especially Lemanja)!

6 TUESDAY

7 WEDNESDAY

8 THURSDAY

Tonight is where you get to take that last pause before the new cycle begins. Where you get to clear and cleanse and release any last fragments of what you have been holding on to.

What can you let go of tonight?

What's in the way of you living your dreams?

What can you release so that you are more supported for the next moon cycle?

As the moon is dark, the stars are brighter with hope, divinity and wisdom – use them tonight, perhaps by sitting outside and gazing at the show they put on for you.

9 FRIDAY ○

The super new moon today falls in the airy sign of Aquarius. Aquarian energy is about giving life, but most importantly it is about allowing this 'flow of life' to fill your cup first to overflowing and then allowing that to flow through you to the rest of your world.

You have been trained to give to everyone else first so when the moon falls in Aquarius you may notice some areas of your life that you have been over-giving to. Make the choice to fill your cup first. No, it's not selfish. I call it empowering and you deserve to feel empowered.

10 SATURDAY

It's a wonderfully auspicious day. You have the new moon shining her lunar energy down on you and the start of the Chinese New Year – the year of the dragon. For an extra sprinkle of luck and auspicious energy, wear red each day this week to call that into your world.

11 SUNDAY

12 MONDAY

13 TUESDAY

As you wake and stretch and feel your way into the beginnings of this moon cycle, notice what you are feeling today. Nah, not what the weather is up to or what is happening around you ... look 'in'.

What am I feeling today?

What is the story of me today?

What do I feel like aiming toward for this moon cycle?

Am I feeling a little loopy and all in my head, disconnected maybe?

This moon is in the airy sign of Aquarius; how can I connect to the earth and nature a tiny bit more to ground my energy in?

14 WEDNESDAY

Happy Valentine's Day, baby. ♥

It's in the space that you hold open your heart and throw your arms wide open to receiving even more love today ... there you will find the magic of this day.

In honoring where you are this year – single, partnered, alone – it doesn't matter, it's all radiantly beautiful.

It's exquisitely loving yourself ALL day with each breath, with every cell of your being.

Love her as much as you can, cause gosh she sooo deserves that!

15 THURSDAY

16 FRIDAY ◖

17 SATURDAY

18 SUNDAY

19 MONDAY

Any twirling as you walk through your day will add extra gold stars toward miracles ... take the twirl, baby!

20 TUESDAY

21 WEDNESDAY

22 THURSDAY

23 FRIDAY

24 SATURDAY ●

Today's full moon falls in Virgo and it is
reminding you that you hold the power
to change your life. Notice the ways you
block or sabotage yourself from being
unapologetically you and explore what's in
the way of you living from a place of trust
and flow, standing in your divine goddess
power and being magnificent you.

25 SUNDAY

26 MONDAY

With those full moon vibes still holding strongly, you are being invited to tune into what you need. From a loving space of kindness and compassion, feel into what needs a tweak; your diet, exercise, your time to connect into your intuition, stillness, your connection to nature or the land using your goddess tools to support you.

Where can you choose what you need even more?

27 TUESDAY

28 WEDNESDAY

29 THURSDAY

Are you ready to take a leap today?

    February 29 opens a powerful energy portal that can help you take big leaps in the direction of your dreams. Get crystal clear on what you are leaping toward and take off like a rocket ship in that direction today! 5, 4, 3, 2, 1 ... BLAST OFF!

1 FRIDAY

2 SATURDAY

3 SUNDAY ◑

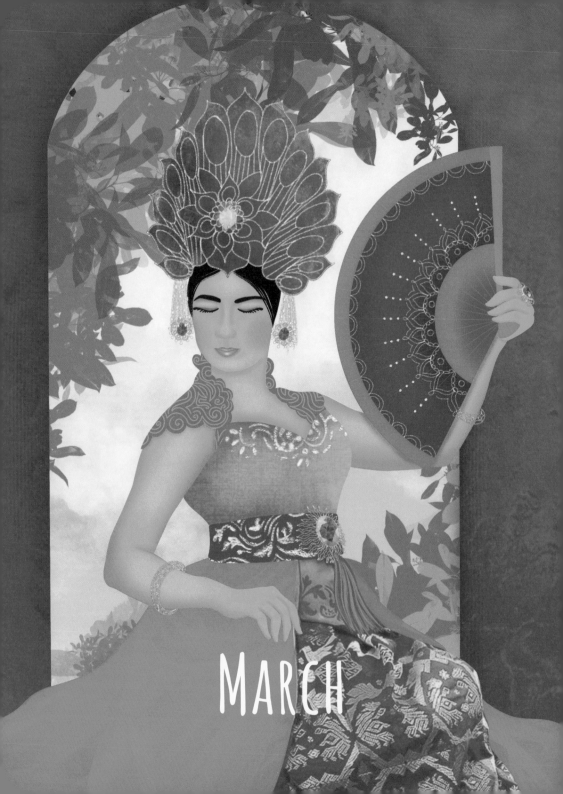

MARCH

DEWI RATIH

Dewi Ratih is a Hindu moon goddess worshipped throughout Indonesia and Bali for her breathtaking beauty and grace. Legend has it that the giant Kala Rau fell desperately and completely in love with *her as she was the most beautiful of all the goddesses; however, Dewi Ratih did not love him back and refused to marry him.* Enraged, Kala Rau tried to steal a drink of the gods to give himself immortality so he could pursue and win her over. But his plan was discovered and the King of the Gods, Dewa Wisnu, went after him to cut off his head with his magical disc. He was too late as the elixir of immortality had reached his throat, making Kala Rau's head immortal.

Dewi Ratih is forever chased by the head of Kala Rau; when he catches her and eats her whole, a lunar eclipse occurs. She slips out of his neck, restoring light to the world and continuing to spread her light and magic across the night sky.

She has come through to support you this month so that when drama is chasing you and you become swallowed by the darkness, you too can call on her to support you to become rebirthed. You can stand in your radiant light sprinkling your magic and your medicine throughout your life and the whole world and you can learn to trust that life supports you.

Dewi Ratih's mantra is 'I am learning to trust that I am safe in this breath and in this moment.'

Her crystals are gold and Burmese rubies for the vital life-force flowing through your body.

Her totem is a hand-held painted fan for flaming her desires and warding off evil.

Her exercises are aerials, acrobatics, pole-dancing and silks to stay bendy and strong.

Her scents are deep scents such as incense sticks (nag-champa), orchid and pine.

4 MONDAY

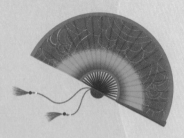

5 TUESDAY

Dewi Ratih asks you to set a timer for five minutes then close your eyes and get comfortable. As you find your stillness, she holds her fan in her hand and is warding off the next layer of any negative energy surrounding your body ... keep breathing that all out.

Now she will dance over your body and use her fan's graceful movements to fan the flames of your desires, to turn them up to make them more vital, alive, expanded and strong ... breathe all that in.

I wonder what you will be guided to move toward today.

6 WEDNESDAY

7 THURSDAY

8 FRIDAY

The dark nights of the waning moon are a time of such sacredness and magic. This lead-up to the new moon birthing brings you this gift of beautiful, mystical nights which hold the space for you to let go of anything you have been holding on to, allowing it to dissolve away. It's like a surrendering to all that is going on in your life right now, a softening into acceptance and love. A pause. How can you rest more over the next few days?

9 SATURDAY

10 SUNDAY ○

Happy Mother's Day, UK! Connect with today's new supermoon in Pisces. Feel her rays shine down into your body igniting healing and awareness. What is she whispering to you?

She is reminding you of your gifts, your talents, your magic. You are a sacred part of this world. You matter. You are guided. You just ... belong.

11 MONDAY

12 TUESDAY

13 WEDNESDAY

Just one more week to use all the tools you have chosen in your winter goddess self-care toolkit. Dance, cook, smell, wear your crystal, call in your goddess and soak up those last fragments of support throughout your week.

14 THURSDAY

15 FRIDAY

I mean if you truly understood just how beautiful and special you actually were, you'd never doubt that you could light up your life with your joy, your giggles or the twinkle in your eyes when you feel connected and alive. Shine and sparkle your light today, baby!

16 SATURDAY

As winter draws to a close and the seasons begin to shift, where are you being called to adventure this weekend? Inside. Outside. A gallery. Skiing. The museum. Shopping. A friend's house. A date.

Gosh, so many options and places to sprinkle your light in.

17 SUNDAY ◑

18 MONDAY

Pop aside some sacred minutes this week to do your goddess self-care toolkit for spring. Make the time to choose what you need to support you through the season as the season makes this time to weave in extra magic for you, too. And you are always down for extra magic, hey (wink wink)!

19 TUESDAY

20 WEDNESDAY

Ahhhh the new light of the season begins to sprinkle down her magic and potency throughout your land today. The spring equinox or Ostara heralds this special day of equal parts day and night, where the light and the shadow are balanced.

This new light signifies balance, harmony and shaking off the winter season with the rebirth into your spring.

Stand outside (or where you can) for five minutes and allow these new rays of sunshine to penetrate through your body, aligning, connecting and balancing your whole being to this new light.

Receive the magic of this ancient celebration.

21 THURSDAY

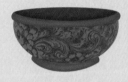

22 FRIDAY

Connect to your new hopes, dreams, desires and wishes for your season ahead. Get clear, write them down and plant the seeds for your intentions in the soil, the land – perhaps dance, drum or sing in your desires.

Clear your space, declutter, wipe down the bench tops, clean the car or burn some incense to intentionally wipe away the winter cobwebs, creating the space to fill it with what you are choosing for spring. With a clearer heart, mind and space, let's dance to your new Goddess toolkit songs together to bring in lots of fresh support for you.

23 SATURDAY

As the energy of the full moon lunar eclipse starts to build, brew and intensify this weekend take a few big breaths, soften your muscles and call yourself into your body, into your now.

Dewi Ratih reminds you to keep your life as simple and nurturing as you can this weekend. She is guiding you through this time. She is with you – that is the gift of using her power and magic to support you. You've so got this, baby.

24 SUNDAY

25 MONDAY ●

Today's full moon and penumbral lunar eclipse falls in the airy sign of Libra. It is a magical time of big shifts, changes, breaking free and 'seeing' what has been hidden from you for a long time. Eclipses open healing portals that push, nudge and help you transcend through outdated ways that are no longer aligned to your soul path.

This time can be deeply uncomfortable in the awareness and the letting go. Remember that the rewards on the other side are always worth the struggle and the pain.

What are you being called to let go of so you may step into the empowered version of yourself?

26 TUESDAY

27 WEDNESDAY

As the charge of the lunar eclipse remains strong this week, imagine Dewi Ratih is sending you a spiral of radiant moonlight magic which flows down into your body. Hold your hands out to your side to receive it fully, taking deep breaths and expanding into the powerful being you truly are and receiving the gift and blessing of exquisite love from her.

28 THURSDAY

29 FRIDAY

Would you like to call in your new spring support team of angels, spirit guides, spirit animals, ancestors and any passed loved ones who will support you this spring to be the most potent, amazing and grounded version of yourself as you start to walk in the direction of your dreams? Do it! Do it! Do it! Call them in, baby!

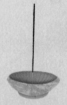

30 SATURDAY

31 SUNDAY

Today opens a beautiful Easter healing gateway of transformation for you. Imagine that a waterfall of light and love is cascading down, through and around your whole body, lighting you up from within. You are so deeply loved, nurtured and held in this healing energy, receive it with your arms open wide.

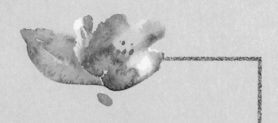

MY GODDESS SELF-CARE TOOLKIT FOR SPRING

Spring is the time to turn your focus outward. It's the phase of gently unfurling your leaves and rebirthing into this season. The weather is warming up, the days start to become longer and the flowers begin to bloom.

Set your intentions for the next 12 weeks, which will be a time for you to see your magic and to sparkle brighter. This is also a great time for clearing clutter, a perfect time to wear some bright-colored clothing, a special time to journal, and a time for taking walks through nature and observing the changes happening all around you.

Have a look back at the toolkit you created for winter and note how it has supported you. Did you use all your tools to their full potential or does something need a little adjustment? Send each of your tools a big heartfelt thank you for supporting you through the last season.

All the self-care tools you choose here will support you from today until the summer solstice in June. These self-care tools will help you shine through your spring season with extra sprinkles of love and magic.

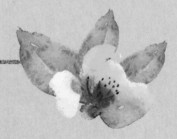

GODDESS MEDICINE

Let's start with choosing a goddess. Flip through until you come to April, May and June. Really notice the picture of each goddess and read the description about her. Which goddess feels like she will help you the most this season? The goddess I have chosen to support me throughout spring 2024 is:

_____

She will support me with the medicine of her

_____

COLOR MEDICINE

Choose one color that is going to support you throughout spring. Land on your color and write it down here:

_____

When I see this color, I feel

_____

I can use this color to support me throughout spring with things such as clothing, accessories, jewelry, flowers, scatter cushions, candles, crystals, pens and

_____

SOUND MEDICINE

Choose three songs. Songs that you love, songs that get you up and moving, songs that make you feel that it's impossible to stay completely still, songs that make you feel like you want to boom-shakka-lakka and shimmy-shake around your house. When you feel irritated, what could you do to get those deep irritations and emotions out of your body? You can dance them out! Yes, I know it sounds a little bit weird (okay, super weird) but it really does work. If I am feeling a little triggered, angry, scared, irritated or just in a funk, I can play these three songs so I can get all loose and not caring, and allow the music and dance to move me through the emotion.

My three songs are:

1. _____

2. _____

3. _____

Your song mission is to download your three songs and create a special spring playlist on your phone so that, whenever you need them, they are ready for you.

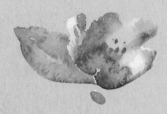

BODY MOVEMENT MEDICINE

Moving your body is important: you know that, I know that, everyone knows that. If there was a magical place that you could visit and it would transform your body with the push of a button, we'd all go there, right? Unfortunately, I am yet to discover this place so, for now, we all have to move our bodies to keep them strong, healthy and bendy in the ways we have available to us at this moment. Choose an exercise that feels as joyful, pleasurable, enlightening and as fun as it can be. There are so many ways to move your body. Choose one that feels exciting for you now.

The ways I will move my body during spring are:

_____

I will do these at _____ (location), _____ times per week.

PLANT MEDICINE

Botanicals have been used for thousands of years to support us to stay healthy and strong. Using different plants, their flowers or their fruit to cure ailments, support you to sleep better, help you to feel more vital, boost your immunity, encourage your digestive system to function easier, balance your hormones or help you feel more energized makes you feel like you are supporting your well-being.

Choose one health focus for spring. Write it here:

_____

Now research your focus and commit to taking or using this plant medicine each day throughout spring. You can find so many ways to bring in the magic of plants like supplements, teas, tinctures, essences, rubs or even a fresh bunch of herbs. Remember that tablets, teas, and so on don't work if they stay in the cupboard, they need to be used!

AROMATHERAPY MEDICINE

Your nose is a powerful tool. When you smell something you love, your whole body feels so happy. It is like your nose holds this secret power to connect you to what brings you pleasure. You may even have memories triggered by your sense of smell. In choosing to notice these scents you love and by sprinkling them throughout your day, you will trigger a pleasure response that reminds you to feel all loved up and amazing. Kinda cool, hey! For spring, choose one smell that is going to support you throughout this season. It could be an essential oil, a perfume, a flower. Choose something you just love that is easy to use and fills you with pleasure.

Land on your fragrance and write it down here:

_____

When your nostrils are tickled with this fragrance, how do you feel?

_____

I can use this fragrance as my signature spring scent to support me in lots of ways such as burning essential oils and candles, using in skincare, eating or cooking with it, wearing the perfume, smelling fresh flowers, as well as

_____ and _____

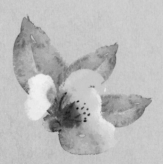

CRYSTAL MEDICINE

Crystals are like magical particles that hold healing powers within. There are thousands of crystals available and they all have individual characteristics or ways to support you. Using the magic of one crystal helps to guide you with what you are working on, with healing, clearing or reminding you how you are growing and what you are wanting to step into. The crystal I am choosing to support me for spring is called

_____

It is _____ (color) and it will help me to

I can use this crystal to support me in lots of ways, such as carrying a piece in my pocket, or keeping a piece in the car or my bag. I could wear it in jewelry, use it as a screensaver on my phone, pop it under my pillow or mattress to support me while I sleep, or I could

_____ or _____

For an extra gold star for being amazing, fill in three things you love most about spring.

1. _____

2. _____

3. _____

I will choose to do these things more because they bring me pleasure and fill my heart with joy. I deserve joy. (Yes, you really do!) Well done. That is your very own goddess self-care toolkit for spring all finished and completed. It will be here to support you through to the summer solstice in June. Call in your goddess and play your three songs now, swaying those hips as you dance and twirl around in celebration of completing your toolkit and being so special.

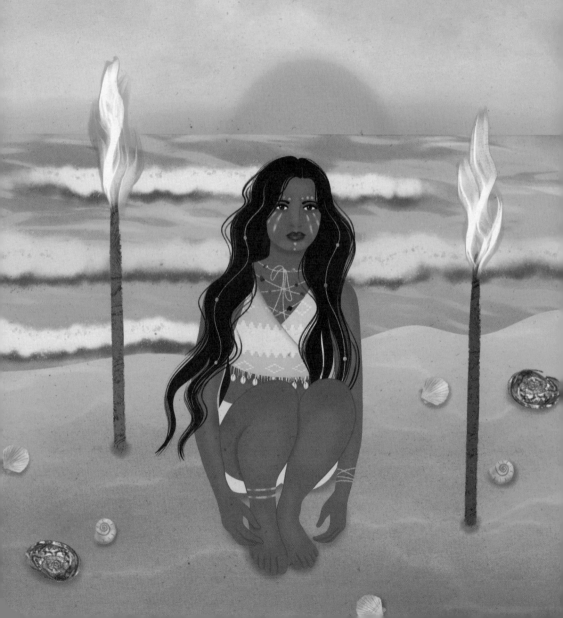

APRIL

YOLKAI ESTSAN

Yolkai Estsan is a beautiful Native American Navajo goddess of the moon and the sea who was fondly known as 'White Shell Woman'. Legend has it that Yolkai Estsan was created by her sister Estsanatlehi out of an abalone shell and cradled in rainbows, which is how she received this sacred name.

Yolkai Estsan has links to the earth and magic, to the sacred cycles of the seasons, and is the great and honored protector of the ocean. She is credited with creating fire and she brings through this month for you the sacred fire element for transformation and courage.

Yolkai Estsan says 'I send you the fire element to burn away your fears, to bring courage to your heart so you may pursue your dreams, to clear your doubts and ignite the flames of your passions and fiery spirit and to help you to transform and feel inspired once more.'

Yolkai Estsan's mantra is 'I am learning to unleash my passion and "burn away" what no longer supports me.'

Her crystals are carnelian and clear quartz.

Her totems are connecting to the great powers of the majestic eagle and abalone shells.

Her exercises are sports involving the land and the sea.

Her scents are fiery, such as pepper, chili and grapefruit.

1 MONDAY

_____

2 TUESDAY ◑

_____

3 WEDNESDAY

_____

4 THURSDAY

Yolkai Estsan sends you an abalone shell to hold you with the highest protection available
to you as you move through your week. Feel yourself standing, held in this protective shell's
warmth, grace, power and courage as you move through the eclipse gateways.

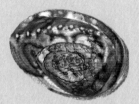

5 FRIDAY

In the lead-up to the total solar eclipse on Monday, you may find yourself (or others) getting
a little stirred up, out of sorts, or feeling argumentative, tired, irritated or just 'over it' all. Be
gentle with yourself and those around you during this time. Your awareness of what is going on
for you is key – use your goddess self-care toolkit to support you through this time.

6 SATURDAY

7 SUNDAY

8 MONDAY ○

Today brings you a total solar eclipse and new supermoon in the fiery sign of Aries – the leader. A solar eclipse is where the moon covers the sun and darkens its surface, intensifying the depth of what is coming into your awareness.

What are you feeling today? How can you lean into the darkness, the shadows and discern what is coming up for you? Such great wonders can be found in your depths. Wisdom and insight are two such treasures. What else will you discover when you go 'in'?

9 TUESDAY

10 WEDNESDAY

II THURSDAY

Your body, your emotions, your mind and your soul are still becoming aligned to the shifts of the solar eclipse and the new moon.

Be kind today and through your week because you, me and everyone is processing, aligning and refining ... like a beautiful bottle of red wine.

Use this energy to love yourself and those around you with patience and extra doses of love medicine blended with a scoop of support. Be gentle with that beautiful one who gazes back at you from the mirror; she really is so amazing.

12 FRIDAY

13 SATURDAY

14 SUNDAY

15 MONDAY ◑
_____

16 TUESDAY
_____

17 WEDNESDAY
_____

18 THURSDAY

19 FRIDAY

Yolkai Estsan sends you this sacred mission: set a timer on your phone for three minutes, close your eyes and just breathe deeply and fully.

Breathe in the support from the earth, the trees, the air, the water, the fire ... all the elements of nature and breathe out any tightness or contraction felt in your body.

For those three minutes today come back to you. Don't overthink it and there's no need to overachieve. Give yourself a tick and then go be all fabulous knowing that for today you have achieved great things.

20 SATURDAY

21 SUNDAY

22 MONDAY

23 TUESDAY

24 WEDNESDAY ●

Happy full moon in the watery sign of Scorpio, beautiful one. As you twirl and move into your day, the moon is radiating her moonbeams of love all over your body and your life. Feel that love!

Scorpio goes into the depths of what you are feeling and uncovers truths, wisdom and insights that have lay buried for years. Listen to those intuitive feelings you will have during this moon and trust yourself more. It is a beautiful time to cleanse your body, mind and soul with the water element, letting go of anything that no longer serves your highest path.

25 THURSDAY

Yolkai Estsan reminds you that you have at your disposal, the medicine and magical energy of the element of water. Use it by skinny dipping, wandering through a creek, beach strolls, sunsets over the water, baths filled with bubbles, mermaiding, pool swims, rain dancing, waterfalls, shell necklaces, surrounding yourself with larimar and moonstones – so, so many nurturing ways to be around water. Which one will you choose to support you this week?

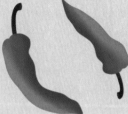

26 FRIDAY

27 SATURDAY

28 SUNDAY

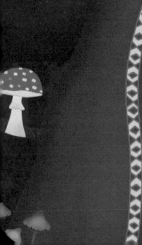

May

DEVANA

Devana is a Slavic goddess of the moon, of wildlife, hunting and fertility. She was fondly known as 'Mother of the Forest'. Devana walks through the forest with a wolf by her side carrying a candle and protecting all the wildlife. She was also tasked with protecting the crops from the freezing temperatures that could cause them to perish in Russia and Poland.

Legend has it that on the change of the seasons, a sacred tree would be beautifully decorated and adorned with special objects, and songs would be sung by her worshippers as they called in the change of the seasons. The sacred tree was called May. What a perfect month for Devana to support you through!

Each spring Devana would take a sacred ritual bath in a body of water to signify her being reborn: refreshed and renewed and reconnected to her divine feminine powers. She has a wild and free spirit that flows through her, and this is what she brings to you this month – a reconnection to you being untamed, wild and free.

Devana's mantra is 'I am learning to live untamed and reconnect to my wild and free nature.'

Her crystals are ambers, resins and woods – gifts from the forest.

Her totems are wolves for connecting to the power of the moon and a bow and arrow for hunting and protecting the wildlife.

Her exercises are rock climbing and team sports.

Her scents are of the forest: bark, lemon balm, eucalyptus, lemon myrtle and oak.

29 MONDAY

Yolkai Estsan's message for you – 'Today may you take the next tiny step forward. You are learning to unleash your passions and "burn away" what no longer supports you. Change comes when you take action. Take the action, darling.'

30 TUESDAY

I WEDNESDAY ◑

Devana asks you to notice what makes you feel free. How can you give this to yourself in radical ways this week?

2 THURSDAY

_____

3 FRIDAY

_____

4 SATURDAY

_____

5 SUNDAY

_____

6 MONDAY

7 TUESDAY

Tonight's dark night brings you the opportunity to take a last pause before the new moon begins tomorrow. Feeling extra tired is normal around this time in the moon cycle. What do you need to support you from your toolkit? Extra cuddles are always lovely.

8 WEDNESDAY ○

Today brings you the beginning of the next moon cycle. It's a new moon in the earthy sign of Taurus and a wonderful time for you to start feeling into what you would like to achieve during this moon cycle.

It's an expansive time with vast possibilities, so much more is possible for you so keep stretching into your desires and choosing what you want. Keep your dreams achievable, fun, sensual ... dreams that feel pleasurable and that fill you up with joy sprinkles. Feel into the whispers of your inner knowing for it is heightened under this moon.

9 THURSDAY

10 FRIDAY

11 SATURDAY

12 SUNDAY

Happy Mother's Day, America! To all the moms who nurture and love their children, fur babies, plants, family, friends, nieces, cousins and neighbors. Your exquisite love is so needed and valued. Thank you for your belief in the possibilities and dreams of those around you. You change the world.

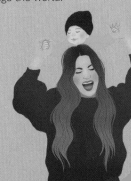

13 MONDAY

Devana reminds you to notice how much you have changed, learnt and grown as a whole being recently. What have you learnt and how can you use these learnings to empower you to keep breaking free of any cages you feel trapped in? Wild and free, baby ... it's time.

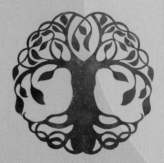

14 TUESDAY

15 WEDNESDAY ◑

16 THURSDAY

17 FRIDAY

18 SATURDAY

Devana reminds you how much wilder
and freer you feel when you choose
simplicity, play, connection to Mother Earth,
sustainability and love ... while deeply
honoring yourself. That way you'll always feel
more fabulous and more you, and you are so
cute when you honor yourself.

19 SUNDAY

20 MONDAY

21 TUESDAY

22 WEDNESDAY

23 THURSDAY ●

What cool energy you have available to you as you land firmly in the full moon vibes today. Happy full moon, baby! Sagittarius is the fiery sign of passions, adventures and doing things with a sense of edginess. You may be feeling fired up about something, angry, powerless, discontented or just sick of dragging baggage around with you. Stomp out the irritations into the earth.

How can you give to yourself, love yourself, trust yourself even more passionately during this moment? Devana reminds you that you deserve your dreams, those wild and free ones this year, so choose them today.

24 FRIDAY

25 SATURDAY

26 SUNDAY

27 MONDAY

28 TUESDAY

29 WEDNESDAY

30 THURSDAY ◑

Devana invites you to take a sacred ritual bath with her, signifying your rebirth into spring, feeling refreshed, renewed and reconnected to your divine feminine powers.

Immerse your whole body in water – the ocean, a lake, a pool, your bathtub or shower. Call in and ask to connect to Devana; don't overthink it, just trust you've got this and allow the water to flow over you, cleansing and resetting all the cycles in your body.

As you exit the bath, stand proudly with an open heart, reborn, refreshed and ready to be you with a new foundation of your sacred feminine and sexual prowess.

31 FRIDAY

1 SATURDAY

2 SUNDAY

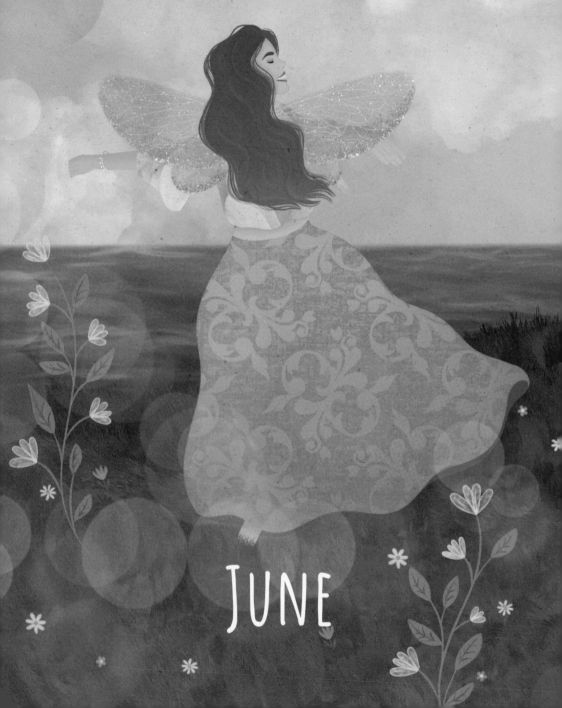

AINE

Aine is an Irish goddess of the moon, of love and the harvest. She is known as 'The Faery Queen' — a faery goddess, yes please! Aine has a beautiful playful nature, she is young and filled with joy. She loves being outdoors in the hills and loughs of Ireland and she just loves the smell and the feel of summer. June in Ireland is Aine's favorite time of the year, so she is your perfect moon goddess for this month.

Aine was an incredible healer and diviner of magic who has been worshipped for supporting people (especially women) to bring in luck, good fortune, fertility and abundance. According to ancient myths, through Aine's playful nature and loving ways she birthed the faery race into reality and has been known as the queen of the faery's ever since.

Aine encapsulates joy-filled bubbles of luminescent light that fill her body and as she fills up so much with all the things that she loves, she sends them out into the world to support others. She is so much like the playful faeries from books when you were young.

Aine's mantra is 'I am learning to wear my faery wings while playing and filling my body with bubbles of love.'

Her crystals are green ones of the meadows: aventurine, calcite, moss-agate, amazonite and malachite.

Her totems are rabbits for fertility, red mares, swans and onions for protection and warding off evil.

Her exercises are playing freely in some way such as dancing, running, walking, wandering and twirling.

Her scents are herbaceous and fungi such as meadowsweet, blackberry, mistletoe, angelica and mugwort.

3 MONDAY

4 TUESDAY

5 WEDNESDAY

It's a time for retreating right now, so let go of being overly responsible for everyone and everything else. Firm up your boundaries so you can retreat and then rise tomorrow reborn as the sexy, beautiful goddess you are.

6 THURSDAY ○

Today's new moon falls in the airy sign of Gemini, the sign of your mind and intellect. Try to notice where you are feeling overwhelmed or like the same thoughts are running through your mind repeatedly. Journaling these thoughts could help you.

This moon is about how you express yourself in the world. What parts of you have been hidden away for too long now? What is preparing itself to be birthed from you: ideas, projects, changes? What do you need from your toolkit today to feel like you can settle in, soften and allow the changes to flow?

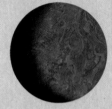

7 FRIDAY

8 SATURDAY

9 SUNDAY

10 MONDAY

Aine is gifting you your very own pair of magical and very sacred faery wings to wear as you work with her more closely this month. Feel those wings placed on your body, they are a perfect fit. Feel the lightness and the playful joy your wings are connecting you to. Maybe you could draw your wings here today.

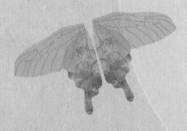

11 TUESDAY

12 WEDNESDAY

13 THURSDAY

14 FRIDAY ◖

If you looked back on what you have achieved during spring what would you notice? Can you see what you have accomplished? Write it down so you can be reminded of what you have done well. Celebrate your success and your amazingness by doing something special for yourself. What will you do or buy, or how could you treat yourself this weekend?

15 SATURDAY

16 SUNDAY

Happy Father's Day to all our amazing dads who sprinkle their loving energy through our world. We love you.

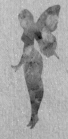

17 MONDAY

Just a few days left before the summer solstice to use your goddess self-care toolkit for spring, squeezing and soaking up those last fragments of support. Play your songs, wear your color, smell your fragrance, move your body and use your crystal energy as much as you can to turn up receiving support. Bathe in the delicious support you have available to you.

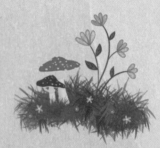

18 TUESDAY

19 WEDNESDAY

With your faery wings firmly in place, Aine by your side and perhaps your goddess toolkit songs playing, could you twirl, dance and radiate out faery magic through your world today? I wonder what you will create when you believe in your magic dancing.

    Keep your eyes open for it, baby, it's there.

20 THURSDAY

21 FRIDAY

Today is the summer solstice, a day that begins the new cycle of the sun's potent energy. It's a chance to really connect to the life force and flames of the sun as it reaches its highest point in the sky.

Watch the sunrise and feel the rays of this new light begin their journey, sit and meditate as the sun sets for the day, or safely bask for five delicious minutes in the sun feeling her heat penetrate through your body.

Stay on the lookout for faeries as this was the day in ancient times they would show themselves to humans ... so cool!

22 SATURDAY

Today that beautiful ball of light in your sky will turn and reach her fullness and brightest illumination for a powerful full moon in the earth sign of Capricorn.

Capricorn is the sign of stability and being grounded. While these qualities may feel a little out of reach over the next few days, trust that what is coming up for you is just perfect for right now.

23 SUNDAY

24 MONDAY

Time to do your new goddess self-care toolkit this week – jump over now and let's do this!

25 TUESDAY

26 WEDNESDAY

27 THURSDAY

28 FRIDAY

Aine is curious to know all about your new tools that you have chosen to support you through this summer season. She lovingly sits waiting to hear all about them. What can you tell her? Why do you love them? Can you play her your songs as you both dance together with your faery wings on?

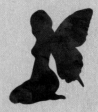

29 SATURDAY

30 SUNDAY

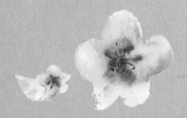

MY GODDESS SELF-CARE TOOLKIT FOR SUMMER

Summer is the time for expanding your energy outward, catching up with friends, feeling the sun's rays on your body and spreading your joy and magic throughout your world.

Set your intentions for the next 12 weeks, which will be a time for you to honor your space, set your boundaries and a great time for choosing your pleasure. This is a time for summer love, toes in the sand, barbecues, picnics and ocean swims.

Have a look back at the toolkit you created for spring and note how it has supported you. Did you use all of your tools to their full potential or does something need a little adjustment? Send each of your tools a big heartfelt thank you for supporting you through the last season.

You outgrow things that support you because you are always changing and growing and shifting. You will find yourself choosing different tools to support you for this season.

All the self-care tools you choose here will support you from today until the fall equinox at the end of September. These self-care tools will help you shine through your summer season with extra sprinkles of love and magic.

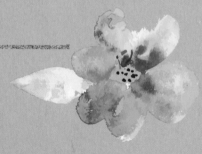

GODDESS MEDICINE

Let's start with choosing a goddess. Flip through until you come to July, August and September. Really notice the picture of each goddess and read the description about her. Which goddess feels like she will help you the most this season? The goddess I have chosen to support me throughout summer 2024 is:

_____

She will support me with the medicine of her

_____

COLOR MEDICINE

Choose one color that is going to support you throughout summer. Land on your color and write it down here:

_____

When I see this color, I feel

_____

I can use this color to support me throughout summer with things such as clothing, accessories, jewelry, flowers, scatter cushions, candles, crystals, pens and

_____

SOUND MEDICINE

Choose three songs. Songs that you love, songs that get you up and moving, songs that make you feel that it's impossible to stay completely still, songs that make you feel like you want to boom-shakka-lakka and shimmy-shake around your house. When you feel irritated, what could you do to get those deep irritations and emotions out of your body? You can dance them out! Yes, I know it sounds a little bit weird (okay, super weird) but it really does work. If I am feeling a little triggered, angry, scared, irritated or just in a funk, I can play these three songs so I can get all loose and not caring, and allow the music and dance to move me through the emotion.

My three songs are:

1. _____

2. _____

3. _____

Your song mission is to download your three songs and create a special summer playlist on your phone so that, whenever you need them, they are ready for you.

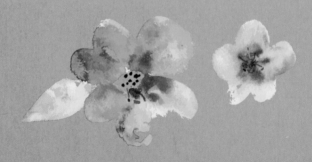

BODY MOVEMENT MEDICINE

Moving your body is important: you know that, I know that, everyone knows that. If there was a magical place that you could visit and it would transform your body with the push of a button, we'd all go there, right? Unfortunately, I am yet to discover this place so, for now, we all have to move our bodies to keep them strong, healthy and bendy in the ways we have available to us at this moment. Choose an exercise that feels as joyful, pleasurable, enlightening and as fun as it can be. There are so many ways to move your body. Choose one that feels exciting for you now.

The ways I will move my body during summer are:

_____

I will do these at _____ (location), _____ times per week.

PLANT MEDICINE

Botanicals have been used for thousands of years to support us to stay healthy and strong. Using different plants, their flowers or their fruit to cure ailments, support you to sleep better, help you to feel more vital, boost your immunity, encourage your digestive system to function easier, balance your hormones or help you feel more energized makes you feel like you are supporting your well-being.

Choose one health focus for summer. Write it here:

_____

Now research your focus and commit to taking or using this plant medicine each day throughout summer. You can find so many ways to bring in the magic of plants like supplements, teas, tinctures, essences, rubs or even a fresh bunch of herbs. Remember that tablets, teas, and so on don't work if they stay in the cupboard, they need to be used!

AROMATHERAPY MEDICINE

Your nose is a powerful tool. When you smell something you love, your whole body feels so happy. It is like your nose holds this secret power to connect you to what brings you pleasure. You may even have memories triggered by your sense of smell. In choosing to notice these scents you love, and by sprinkling them throughout your day, you will trigger a pleasure response that reminds you to feel all loved up and amazing. Kinda cool, hey!

For summer, choose one smell that is going to support you throughout this season. It could be an essential oil, a perfume or a flower. Choose something you just love that is easy to use and fills you with pleasure.

Land on your fragrance and write it down here:

_____

When your nostrils are tickled with this fragrance, how do you feel?

_____

I can use this fragrance as my signature summer scent to support me in lots of ways such as burning essential oils and candles, using in skincare, eating or cooking with it, wearing the perfume, smelling fresh flowers, as well as

_____ and _____

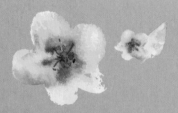

CRYSTAL MEDICINE

Crystals are like magical particles that hold healing powers within. There are thousands of crystals available and they all have individual characteristics or ways to support you. Using the magic of one crystal helps to guide you with what you are working on, with healing, clearing or reminding you how you are growing and what you are wanting to step into.

The crystal I am choosing to support me for summer is called

_____

It is _____ (color) and it will help me to

I can use this crystal to support me in lots of ways, such as carrying a piece in my pocket, or keeping a piece in the car or my bag. I could wear it in jewelry, use it as a screensaver on my phone, pop it under my pillow or mattress to support me while I sleep, or I could

_____ or _____

For an extra gold star for being amazing, fill in three things you love most about summer.

1. _____

2. _____

3. _____

I will choose to do these things more because they bring me pleasure and fill my heart with joy. I deserve joy. (Yes, you really do!) Well done. That is your very own goddess self-care toolkit for summer all finished. It will be here to support you through to the fall equinox in September. Call in your goddess and play your three songs now, swaying those hips as you dance and twirl around in celebration of completing your toolkit and being so special.

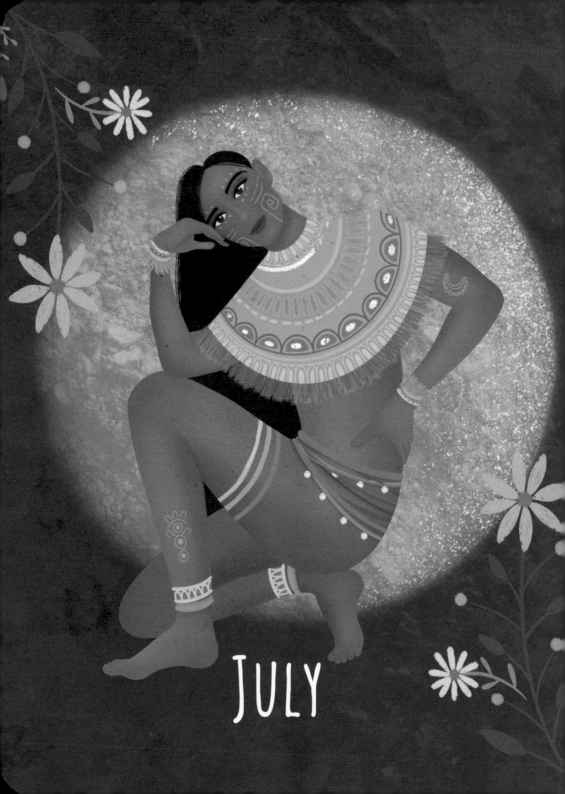

JULY

COYOLXAUHQUI

Coyolxauhqui (pronounced Coy-yo-shar-ki) is honored throughout Mexico, and she is a powerful, radiant and fascinating Aztec moon goddess to learn about. According to legend her dismembered head was thrust up into the skies by her brother Huitzilopochtli and she therefore became the moon.

Coyolxauhqui's medicine for you is the most incredible example of how to turn your greatest traumas, wounds, pain and the drama that can happen in your life into your greatest strength and power, as she does each night by beaming her light across the world and shining as brightly as the moon.

Each moon cycle Coyolxauhqui moves through the cycles of birth, growth, expansion, demise and death. She is here to teach you how to do this in your life too.

Coyolxauhqui's mantra is 'I am learning to alchemize my story of pain into my greatest power.'

Her crystals are fire opal and obsidian for transmuting pain into power.

Her totem is bells, for calling in your magic (she was known as the woman with bells on her face).

Her exercises are sailing across the sea, windsurfing, kitesurfing, gliding and skydiving.

Her scents are of the air, such as lemon, lavender, eucalyptus, may chang and tea tree.

I MONDAY

2 TUESDAY

3 WEDNESDAY

Remember that as the moon darkens you can allow the darkness in so that you see what has been hiding in the shadows for a while now.

What can you let go of in the next few days?

What's in the way of you living your dreams?

What can you release so that you are more supported for the next moon cycle?

4 THURSDAY

What would you like to write a declaration of independence from? An emotion, a person, a habit, a belief perhaps that is holding you back. Where are you feeling the need to be free in your life right now?

I _____ (insert name) am claiming independence from _____ on 4 July 2024. I stand proudly here today, empowered and in a state of flow and grace as I learn how to support myself even more this month.

Twirl that in as you move boldly through your day.

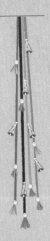

5 FRIDAY ○

Today's gorgeous new moon falls in the watery sign of Cancer, the sign of the divine feminine whose ruling planet is the moon. She is holding the space for you to connect to her insights and wisdom for what feels like home to you.

Nurture and love yourself so much this weekend that your cup is filled first before you heal those around you. What do you need today from your goddess toolkit to support you?

6 SATURDAY

7 SUNDAY

8 MONDAY

Coyolxauhqui sends you this mantra – 'I am learning to alchemize my story of pain into my greatest power.'

    Write it out below in your own handwriting. Say it three times. Know each moment when you decide this to be true it is a deeper connection to your power.

9 TUESDAY

10 WEDNESDAY

11 THURSDAY

12 FRIDAY

13 SATURDAY ◑

14 SUNDAY

15 MONDAY

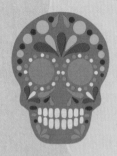

16 TUESDAY

17 WEDNESDAY

Coyolxauhqui moves her head with grace and purpose as she dances around your body today. Can you hear her bells ringing in your passion? Calling to your magic? Connecting you to your medicine? Clearing the way forward for your dreams?

I can!

18 THURSDAY

19 FRIDAY

20 SATURDAY

21 SUNDAY ●

Today's gorgeous full moon in Capricorn and Goddess Coyolxauhqui are helping you be brave and look inside yourself. Look at your own measures of success, your rules and restrictions – are these still aligned with who you are today? Redefine them.

22 MONDAY

Stay present and open to seeing what unfolds for you in the next few days. It's a time for change, for you to do things differently. You are gifted this beautiful time to explore, to clear and cleanse, and to move into a deeper connection with yourself and your relationship to power, money and control.

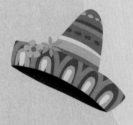

23 TUESDAY

24 WEDNESDAY

25 THURSDAY

26 FRIDAY

27 SATURDAY

Summer weekend magic. How can you
give yourself the gift of a summer weekend
filled with even more things you love about
summer? Ice creams, gelatos, cocktails,
bikinis, beach days?

Now go create that for yourself.

28 SUNDAY

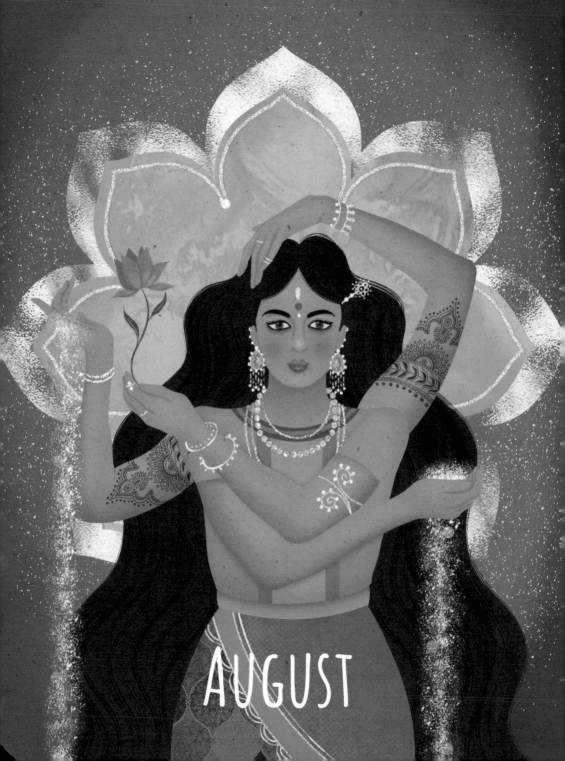

AUGUST

LAKSHMI

Lakshmi is one of my favorite goddesses to work with. She is revered across India and Sri Lanka as the goddess of wealth and abundance. Lakshmi is opulence. She is opulent in gold, jewels and all material possessions, but her true opulence, her most valuable jewels are found inside herself: her inner knowing and wisdom.

She is often represented with four arms signifying the four principals of Hinduism: Dharma – to do one's duty, Artha – the pursuit of wealth, Kama – to feel love, and Moksha – to know oneself.

While not a traditional goddess of the moon (as gods held this title) she is celebrated during the festival Diwali, which revolves around the moon each year, so she can definitely be included for you.

Lakshmi's abundance is received by her on all levels – physical, emotional, mental, relationships, love, money, spiritual and esoteric. She is deeply connected to her spirituality and her team of guides and makes her worship a daily practice so she knows and trusts that she is always supported ... and this is her gift to you this month.

Lakshmi's mantra is 'I am learning to stay open to receiving even more abundance today.'

Her crystals are ones of opulence – yellow and blue sapphires, opals, diamonds and gold.

Her totems are lotus flowers for purity, beauty and enlightenment and elephants for water, work and fertility.

Her exercises are resistance training and gardening.

Her scents are sandalwood and citrus-based scents.

29 MONDAY

30 TUESDAY

31 WEDNESDAY

I THURSDAY

Lakshmi welcomes you to August, the month that she is honored to guide you through this year. She sends you golden coins of abundance that will be sprinkled through your life over the next 30 days. Keep your eyes open to find them.

2 FRIDAY

As the moon darkens and retreats, it is the time for stillness and rest. It's for slowing down, softening into acceptance for what is – a pause. How can you honor this time? What do you need from your toolkit to support you this weekend?

3 SATURDAY

4 SUNDAY ○

Hello, Leo new moon, let's play with the energy of you this moon cycle. Leo is a fire sign, the sign of the lion, so this moon is all about you being regal and confidently you. How could you own and celebrate who you are just that smidgey bit more this whole week? Yes, do that!

5 MONDAY

The golden glowy energy of the Leo new moon will link you into the Lion's Gate portal: a powerful healing gateway that is now open and which will grow to its most potent day on 8 August – 8:8.

Allow the courage it is awakening in you to strengthen and grow today.

6 TUESDAY

7 WEDNESDAY

The Lion's Gate portal of 2024 is a beautiful time to sit in meditation, allowing your heart to be opened and a time to connect into your intuition. The veil between dimensions is thin, so be open to Goddess Lakshmi and your spirit guides sending you whispers of support. Allow their wisdom to rain down on your soul and connect firmly into your heart, into your feet and into the path that you are walking. What is your intention for this sacred portal?

8 THURSDAY

The Lion's Gate portal of 2024 has reached its most potent and powerful day and remains open until 12 August. This gateway is a sacred time that has been honored and celebrated for many thousands of years, especially by ancient civilizations.

Feeling tired, a little emotional – out of sorts? These are all side effects of this portal. Take the time to rest and recalibrate over the next four days, so you can take advantage of all that boldness and lion courage being sent your way.

9 FRIDAY

10 SATURDAY

11 SUNDAY

12 MONDAY ◑

13 TUESDAY

Lakshmi's mantra for you this month is – 'I am learning to stay open to receiving even more abundance today.' Therefore, imagine a funnel sitting just above your head that all your abundance flows through into you. How big is it? How wide is it?

   Now Lakshmi asks you to make your funnel 60 times larger, widen and stretch it out so that you can receive even more flow into your body and your life this month.

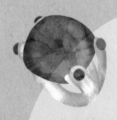

14 WEDNESDAY

15 THURSDAY

16 FRIDAY

17 SATURDAY

18 SUNDAY

19 MONDAY

Today's full moon falls in the airy sign of Aquarius – that beautiful water bearer, the mystical healer that sends water down across the earth healing you, the land and the planet. It's a creative and dreamy energy to work with.

This moon is calling for you to sit under her rays and just be you. Grab your journal, a candle, a crystal, put a playlist on that you love, meditate and moon-bathe under her powerful rays. Create the time to be still, to connect to your support, to dream and to surrender to what is as you look around your life.

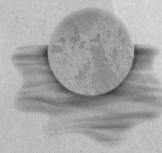

20 TUESDAY

21 WEDNESDAY

22 THURSDAY

23 FRIDAY

24 SATURDAY

25 SUNDAY

26 MONDAY ◗

27 TUESDAY

28 WEDNESDAY

As August draws to a close, look back on your year and notice the ways you have connected to yourself on deeper levels. Spend some time journaling. What did you discover about yourself? When you used your goddess self-care toolkit to support you, how did you feel? What was your greatest achievement each season? Where did you find joy? Where did you find your calm?

Celebrate your success with a little treat this week. You really are so worthy of celebrating.

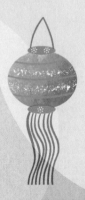

29 THURSDAY

30 FRIDAY

31 SATURDAY

1 SUNDAY

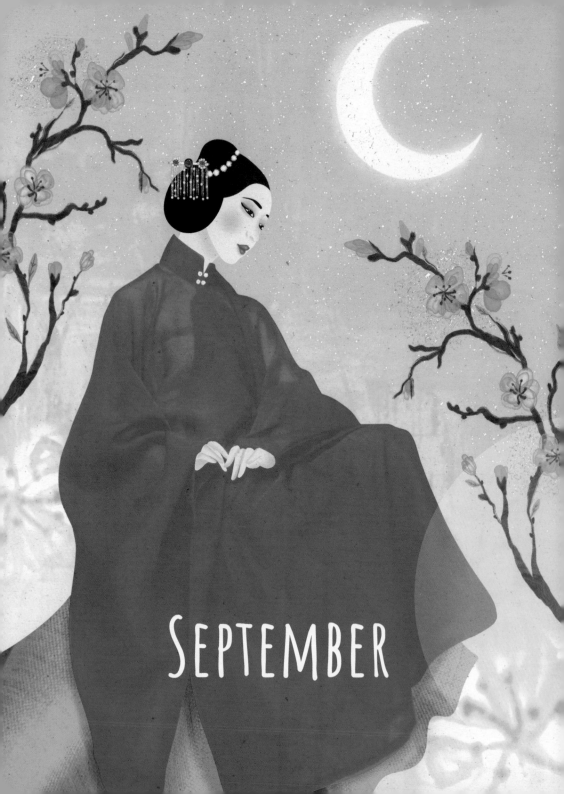

September

CH'ANG-O

Ch'ang-O (Chang'e) is a beautiful and gentle Chinese moon goddess who lives on the moon and is known as 'Woman of the Moon'. According to Chinese mythology, while living in the palace of heaven Ch'ang-O and her handsome husband Hou Yi displeased the Jade Emperor who then banished the couple to earth to live as mortals.

Hou Yi could see that his beautiful wife was miserable in their new life on earth so he went on a quest to discover the pill of immortality, which would make then both immortal once more. Hou Yi located the pill and returned home with it secured in a special case, which he told Ch'ang-O not to touch. Becoming curious Ch'ang-O opened the case and took the whole pill, which was far too much medicine for one person. Ch'ang-O then floated up, up, up into the sky away from her true love Hou Yi. She landed on the moon.

Ch'ang-O was incredibly lonely on the moon waiting for her one true love, so she befriended the Jade Rabbit who she has been mixing elixirs with for over 4000 years (and who you, too, can catch a glimpse of while looking at the moon).

Ch'ang-O has come through to support you this month for the mid-fall or 'Mooncake' festival so that you can learn to receive love in far deeper and more lasting ways.

Ch'ang-O's mantra is 'I am learning to receive love with grace, harmony and an even flow.'

Her crystal is jade for deep wisdom, increasing love and for an extra sprinkle of luck.

Her totems are mooncakes shared with loved ones and lanterns carrying your wishes and dreams to her.

Her exercises are bushwalking, forest bathing and walking in nature collecting herbs.

Her scents are herbaceous such as basil, thyme, lemon balm, rosemary, oregano and coriander.

2 MONDAY

The dark night before the new moon brings you the opportunity to take a last pause before the new moon begins tomorrow. Feeling tired is normal around this time in the moon cycle.
Have you noticed that? Does your bedtime need adjusting tonight? It's a great time for an easy dinner, clearing off your bedside table and having extra water, essential oils and snuggles in bed with a person, pillow, animal or teddy. What do you need today to feel extra supported?

3 TUESDAY ○

As you wake, stretch and feel your way into the beginning of this beautiful new moon cycle, notice with love how you are feeling today. What is the story of you today?

   This moon is in the earthy sign of Virgo; how can you connect to the earth and nature spirits a tiny bit more this moon cycle? What do you need the most to help you do that? How can you prioritize giving that to yourself?

   You really are so very wise when you trust you have the answers you need.

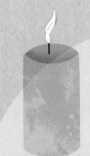

4 WEDNESDAY

5 THURSDAY

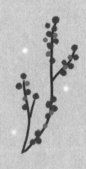

6 FRIDAY

Remember that Ch'ang-O and Mother Earth are with you today, they are helping you to deepen your connection to the sacred earth wisdom and the nature spirits that are dancing in your dreams today.

It's just a thing that they both believe in you. Yep, it just is.

7 SATURDAY

8 SUNDAY

9 MONDAY

If, for this moment, this hour, you chose lightness, joy, pleasure and trusting that life supports you and just breathed that in, I wonder what would change for the rest of your day?

   Oh, do it and let's find out!

10 TUESDAY

11 WEDNESDAY ◑

12 THURSDAY

13 FRIDAY

Today, Friday 13th, is the Day of the Goddess. Tune into your sacred feminine energy today. Wonder at the beauty of you. Nourish your body with moisturizer or spray on an alluring perfume. Light a candle to light up your world with the passion that is you. Flirt with the wind. Drink in the sacred water. Dance through your day on the earth and just radiate your loving medicine everywhere you go.

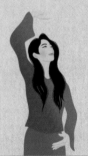

14 SATURDAY

Dancing as you groove through your day will add extra gold stars toward magic happenings swirling through your life ... dance, baby, dance!

15 SUNDAY

16 MONDAY

17 TUESDAY

Ch'ang-O would love to teach you about the Mooncake Festival that is celebrated today. Across China and throughout the world families return home to reunite and reconnect with each other. It is a day filled with stories, connection, sharing an evening meal and worshiping the moon.

Mooncakes are the traditional gift for your loved ones, and they will be shared around the table to celebrate the coming together of family. Kongming lanterns will be decorated and released into the night sky filled with good wishes and thanks to the moon. How could you do a small celebration for the moon and your family on this special day?

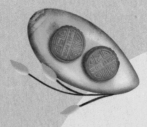

18 WEDNESDAY

Happy supermoon and partial lunar eclipse in Pisces, beautiful one. Can you feel the radiance of your life beaming across the world today? What does that expansion and growth feel like to you today? Where are you feeling the whispers of this eclipse the most in your life; what is she shining her light on for you?

What old stories, over-giving or wounds are you feeling called to release or clear? How can you connect to this beautiful time? What do you need today from your goddess toolkit?

19 THURSDAY

Mermaiding is always a treat around a Pisces full moon; play with the water today!

20 FRIDAY

21 SATURDAY

22 SUNDAY

Today is the fall equinox, a sacred time of seeing the abundance that is sprinkled throughout your life. A healing gateway opens and is an opportunity for you to tap into your intuition on deeper levels, heal imbalances and see your life from a new perspective.

What do you need to notice, feel or hear today to bring more balance back into your life?

23 MONDAY

It's a great time to do your goddess self-care toolkit this week ... flip to the page and let's do this one with the loving waves of Ch'ang-O to help you.

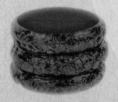

24 TUESDAY ◑

25 WEDNESDAY

26 THURSDAY

Imagine that Ch'ang-O and the Jade Rabbit have created a special potion to support you through the whole fall season. They have filled it with exactly what you most need: infinite, gentle and loving waves of amazing and healing fall grace. Feel the potion flowing down all over and into your body and pouring out through your day to sprinkle extra love as you walk. Oh, how loved you are.

27 FRIDAY

28 SATURDAY

29 SUNDAY

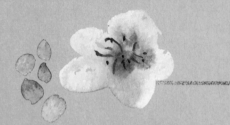

MY GODDESS SELF-CARE TOOLKIT FOR FALL

Fall is the time to turn inward, retreat and enjoy the changes of the season, the weather temperature cooling and the seasonal foods.

Set your intentions for the next 12 weeks, which will be a time for you to honor your space, set your boundaries, and focus on healing and meditation. This is also a perfect time to snuggle in, a time to journal and definitely a time for taking long baths with a fabulous book.

Have a look back at the toolkit you created for summer and note how it has supported you. Did you use your tools to their full potential or does something need a little adjustment? Send each of your tools a big heartfelt thank you for supporting you throughout the summer season.

You outgrow things that support you because you are always changing and growing and shifting. You will find yourself choosing different tools to support you for this season.

All the self-care tools you choose here will support you from today until the winter solstice in December. These self-care tools will help you to shine through your fall season with extra sprinkles of love and magic.

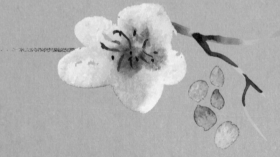

GODDESS MEDICINE

Let's start with choosing a goddess. Flip through until you come to October, November and December. Really notice the picture of each goddess and read the description about her. Which goddess feels like she will help you the most this season? The goddess I have chosen to support me throughout fall 2024 is:

_____

She will support me with the medicine of her

_____

COLOR MEDICINE

Choose one color that is going to support you throughout fall. Land on your color and write it down here:

_____

When I see this color, I feel

_____

I can use this color to support me throughout fall with things such as clothing, accessories, jewelry, flowers, scatter cushions, candles, crystals, pens and

_____

SOUND MEDICINE

Choose three songs. Songs that you love, songs that get you up and moving, songs that make you feel that it's impossible to stay completely still, songs that make you feel like you want to boom-shakka-lakka and shimmy-shake around your house. When you feel irritated, what could you do to get those deep irritations and emotions out of your body? You can dance them out! Yes, I know it sounds a little bit weird (okay, super weird) but it really does work. If I am feeling a little triggered, angry, scared, irritated or just in a funk, I can play these three songs so I can get all loose and not caring, and allow the music and dance to move me through the emotion.

My three songs are:

1. _____

2. _____

3. _____

Your song mission is to download your three songs and create a special fall playlist on your phone so that, whenever you need them, they are ready for you.

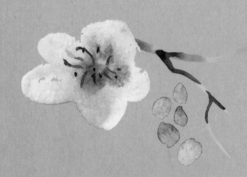

BODY MOVEMENT MEDICINE

Moving your body is important: you know that, I know that, everyone knows that. If there was a magical place that you could visit and it would transform your body with the push of a button, we'd all go there, right? Unfortunately, I am yet to discover this place so, for now, we all have to move our bodies to keep them strong, healthy and bendy in the ways we have available to us at this moment. Choose an exercise that feels as joyful, pleasurable, enlightening and as fun as it can be. There are so many ways to move your body. Choose one that feels exciting for you now.

The ways I will move my body during fall are:

_____

I will do these at _____ (location), _____ times per week.

PLANT MEDICINE

Botanicals have been used for thousands of years to support us to stay healthy and strong. Using different plants, their flowers or their fruit to cure ailments, support you to sleep better, help you to feel more vital, boost your immunity, encourage your digestive system to function easier, balance your hormones or help you feel more energized makes you feel like you are supporting your well-being.

Choose one health focus for fall. Write it here:

_____

Now research your focus and commit to taking or using this plant medicine each day throughout fall. You can find so many ways to bring in the magic of plants like supplements, teas, tinctures, essences, rubs or even a fresh bunch of herbs. Remember that tablets, teas, and so on don't work if they stay in the cupboard, they need to be used!

AROMATHERAPY MEDICINE

Your nose is a powerful tool. When you smell something you love, your whole body feels so happy. It is like your nose holds this secret power to connect you to what brings you pleasure. You may even have memories triggered by your sense of smell. In choosing to notice these scents you love, and by sprinkling them throughout your day, you will trigger a pleasure response that reminds you to feel all loved up and amazing. Kinda cool, hey! For fall, choose one smell that is going to support you throughout this season. It could be an essential oil, a perfume or a flower. Choose something you just love that is easy to use and fills you with pleasure.

Land on your fragrance and write it down here:

_____

When your nostrils are tickled with this fragrance, how do you feel?

_____

I can use this fragrance as my signature fall scent to support me in lots of ways such as burning essential oils and candles, using in skincare, eating or cooking with it, wearing the perfume, smelling fresh flowers, as well as

_____ and _____

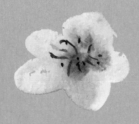

CRYSTAL MEDICINE

Crystals are like magical particles that hold healing powers within. There are thousands of crystals available and they all have individual characteristics or ways to support you. Using the magic of one crystal helps to guide you with what you are working on, with healing, clearing or reminding you how you are growing and what you are wanting to step into.

The crystal I am choosing to support me for fall is called

_____

It is _____ (color) and it will help me to _____

I can use this crystal to support me in lots of ways, such as carrying a piece in my pocket or keeping a piece in the car or my bag. I could wear it in jewelry, use it as a screensaver on my phone, pop it under my pillow or mattress to support me while I sleep, or I could

_____ or _____

For an extra gold star for being amazing, fill in three things you love most about fall.

1. _____

2. _____

3. _____

I will choose to do these things more because they bring me pleasure and fill my heart with joy. I deserve joy. (Yes, you really do!) Well done. That is your very own goddess self-care toolkit for fall all finished. It will be here to support you through to the winter solstice in December. Call in your goddess and play your three songs now, swaying those hips as you dance and twirl around in celebration of completing your toolkit and being so special.

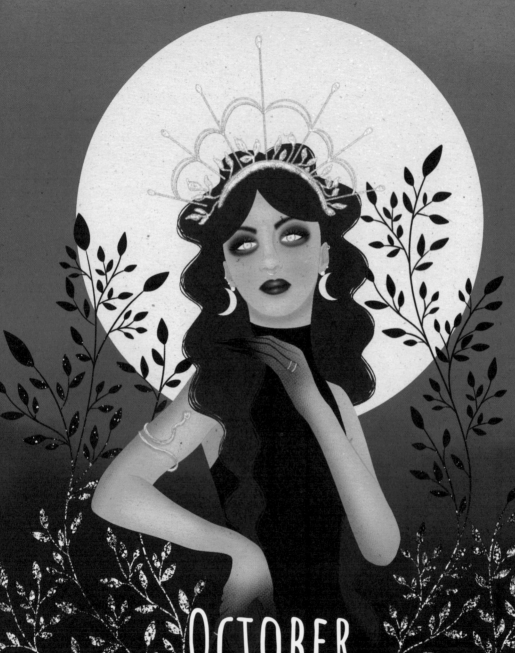

OCTOBER

HECATE

Hecate is the Greek goddess of the moon, of the night and of magic. She is known as the divine mother of all witches. She is often depicted as the Triple Goddess who uses and claims all parts of who she is, or the crone (or wise woman) who is associated with the dark (waning) phase of the moon — one of the most powerful times for magic.

Hecate has this incredible capacity and power to own her many gifts of witchcraft, necromancy (talking to spirits), sorcery, magic, intuition, being the oracle and the healer. One of her gifts is to hold strong connections to both the earth and to the underworld, and she holds the keys to help you access gateways of transformation and entrances to other realms, supporting your growth and sage wisdom.

Hecate holds a vast and deep wisdom inside of her that she uses to transcend between worlds and to weave her magic spells. She is a fierce protector of women and witches on all levels of their divine feminine journey. She is loyal, brave and independent as she weaves magic for her supporters and havoc for those who aren't. She is a beautiful and powerful energy to work with this month.

Hecate's mantra is 'I am learning to create magic in my life.'

Her crystals are moonstone, jasper and obsidian for protection and transmutation.

Her totems are black cauldrons for creating and making magic and silver keys to unlock the gateways to other realms.

Her exercises are running, walking or cycling.

Her scents are of the forest or bush such as bark, trees, resin, fallen leaves and herbs.

30 MONDAY

As you move through this eclipse gateway, Ch'ang-O reminds you of her mantra for you – 'I am learning to receive love with grace, harmony and even flow.' Stay open to receiving support, darling one, for eclipse gateways can be triggering and difficult times. Trust that life does support you to clear, to heal, to grow and to be more exquisitely loved than you even thought possible. Feel the ways of this love flow into your heart and swirl through the rest of your body.

1 TUESDAY

The dark moon phase is one of the most powerful times for magic, therefore Hecate invites you to connect with her in ritual tonight on the dark moon and eclipse gateways.

Light a candle and surround it with some garden herbs that you have on-hand (like rosemary) creating your little altar. Ask for Hecate to join you and write down what your deepest fears are. What has been stirred up with the eclipse? Then wait for her response and write down what you feel she is saying to you. Send her your heartfelt thanks for guiding you tonight and through the month ahead. Blow out your candle to close your ritual.

2 WEDNESDAY ○

Today brings you an airy new moon in Libra and an annular solar eclipse. Today the moon covers the sun darkening its surface, so the depth of what is coming into your awareness and what you 'feel' is intensified.

It marks an incredible opportunity for you to feel into this energy that is nudging you to see with new eyes what is out of balance in your life and the world around you. Breathe deeply, place your hands on your heart and notice what is stirring for you today. What is significant ... notice, baby, because you are meant to see.

3 THURSDAY

4 FRIDAY

5 SATURDAY

It's been a big few weeks with big shifts for you.
What do you need to use from your goddess
self-care toolkit to support you this weekend?

6 SUNDAY

7 MONDAY

8 TUESDAY

9 WEDNESDAY

Hecate asks you to notice where you are creating and weaving magic through your life. It is already happening. You do use your sacred gifts to create magical outcomes for yourself and your loved ones. Notice more this week what you already do. Such power you hold.

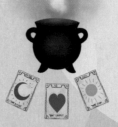

10 THURSDAY ◑

_____

11 FRIDAY

_____

12 SATURDAY

_____

13 SUNDAY

_____

14 MONDAY

Fire up today, baby, from deep within your heart and your belly, call in that fierce warrior strength of Goddess Hecate and the moon to inspire your baby steps forward in the direction of your beautiful, inspired dreams this week.

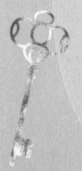

15 TUESDAY

16 WEDNESDAY

17 THURSDAY

It's supermoon day in the fiery sign of Aries. Take a big breath and connect into her energy, her strength, her fullness. Aries is the fire, the fierce motivation, the awakening of your desires, passions and your warrior strength. This full moon is urging you to purge what is no longer in your highest good to carry.

Journal on what you are choosing to release, write it down and burn it (safely) to ashes, scattering away what you are choosing to clear. Sit under this moon, bathing in her rays of moonlight magic and inspiration, creating the space for your dreams to be.

18 FRIDAY

19 SATURDAY

Gosh, what a wonderful time to be alive ... what a wonderful time to be fierce and sexy YOU! Put on your fall playlist of three songs and dance in the sexy factor of you today with Hecate.

20 SUNDAY

21 MONDAY

22 TUESDAY

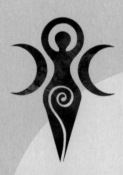

23 WEDNESDAY

24 THURSDAY

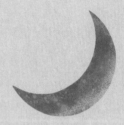

25 FRIDAY

Hecate is sending you a sacred orb of liquid crystal. This orb holds the energetic imprint of the highest level of protection that will surround you for the rest of 2024. It is a perfect infusion of white moonstone to support you to amplify your powers, black obsidian to alchemize negative energy into positive energy and red jasper for knowing that her life blood pumps through your veins; you are connected deeply to her.

Feel this orb surround you fully now and as you move through your day.

26 SATURDAY

27 SUNDAY

28 MONDAY

29 TUESDAY

30 WEDNESDAY

31 THURSDAY

The ancient celebrations of Halloween, Samhain and Day of the Dead all fall over the next few days. However you choose to celebrate, know that the veil between realms is so thinly held right now, your ancestors and your spirit guide team are sending you signs of their presence in your life.

Know that Hecate is sending magical things through your life this year; stay on the lookout for them. Know that blessings of exquisite love are flowing into your life; stay open to receiving them.

Sometimes, the simplest ritual of lighting a candle and sending thanks and gratitude to all those who walk with you and cheer you on in this lifetime is enough. Keep it simple and extra loving.

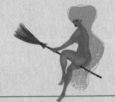

I FRIDAY ○

Today's new moon of transformation and rebirth falls in the watery sign of Scorpio. Use the deep potency of this new moon by standing with your arms open wide to receive her moon dust magical flow, allowing her to support you in your transformation and rebirth. For today, like the phoenix who rises from the ashes, so too shall you.

2 SATURDAY

Happy Day of the Dead or *Dia de los Muertos*. Send your love and heartfelt gratitude out to all your ancestors for guiding you and walking with you this year. Celebrate today all of who you are and honor just how far you've come. Light a candle and say thank you to each of them.

3 SUNDAY

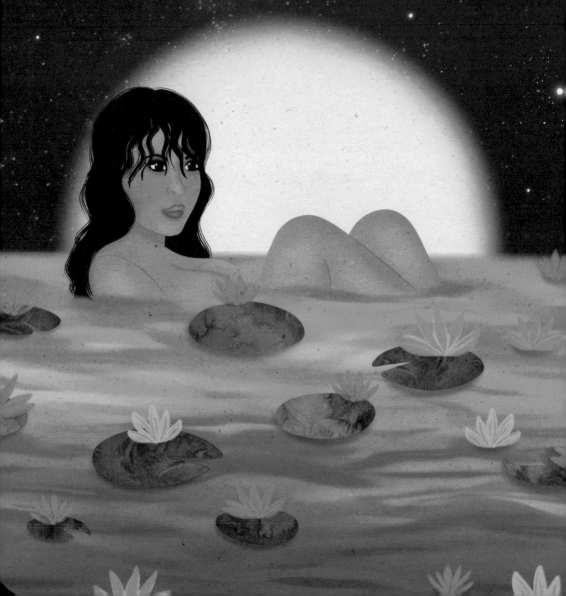

HALIYA

Haliya is the masked goddess of the moon and of moonlight, worshipped in pre-colonial times throughout the Philippines. She symbolizes the strength and potency of women. Haliya is the fierce protector of the moon against the giant sea-serpent-dragon deity Bakunawa who tries to swallow the moon a few times each year (causing lunar eclipses).

Priestesses and wise women would gather in sacred ritual to dance and sing each full moon, circling around a tree and summoning Haliya to protect them from Bakunawa so that light was returned once more to their land.

Haliya and her brother Bulan, the god of the moon, were both incredibly beautiful with luscious dark hair and eyes as dark as midnight. They would travel down to earth and bathe in the freshwater lakes of the Philippines. The moonlight and the beauty from Haliya and Bulan was so radiant that the next day takay flowers would appear from the muddy depths, covering the surface of the lake in bold pinks.

Legend has it that Haliya wore a mask of gold, shielding her incredible beauty from those around her. She has come through to support you this month giving you the courage to stand radiant and proud as the divine being you are. As you learn to embrace the goddess that resides within you, you too can remove your mask and learn to radiate your profound beauty through your world.

Haliya's mantra is 'I am learning to lower my barriers and embrace the beauty of who I am.'

Her crystals are gold, moonstone and amethyst.

Her totems are takay and lotus flowers, for connecting to the beauty of color and nature.

Her exercises are qi-gong, yoga and martial arts to stay strong and supple.

Her scents are alluring, such as lotus flowers, frangipani, ylang-ylang and ginger for spice.

4 MONDAY

5 TUESDAY

6 WEDNESDAY

Haliya says: I send you this mantra to support you through this month. 'I am learning to lower my barriers and embrace the beauty of who I am.' Where can you be one per cent more vulnerable this week?

When you lower your mask and show the radiance of who you are, you shine. Be brave, my darling, for it is in the sharing of who you truly are that the world cannot help but fall in love with you in deeper ways.

7 THURSDAY

_____

8 FRIDAY

_____

9 SATURDAY ◑ _____   10 SUNDAY _____

11 MONDAY

12 TUESDAY

13 WEDNESDAY

14 THURSDAY

15 FRIDAY

Happy full moon, baby. Feel into that energy shift today. This earthy Taurus moon is powerful; she is potent, abundant and expansive with lots of transformational moonbeams flowing down to you. It's a great time to start to curiously explore and feel into what this moon is whispering to you – what are you being called to clear, to release, to remember?

Use the earth element to help you stay stable, strong, connected and grounded into the earth.

16 SATURDAY

17 SUNDAY

18 MONDAY

19 TUESDAY

20 WEDNESDAY

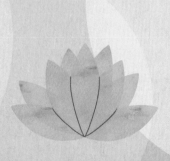

21 THURSDAY

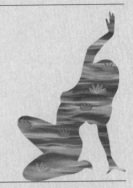

22 FRIDAY

Haliya invites you to bathe in the sacred lakes of the Philippines with her. Imagine that you are standing at the edge of these sacred waters, the moonlight shining down. Look around – what else is there? Stepping into the water with Haliya by your side, you feel so nurtured and held. You are safe here.

Immerse your whole body in the fresh water. Feel it covering you, holding you, nourishing you. Feel your inner beauty radiate out across the lake sprinkling the magic that is needed for the takay flowers to blossom tomorrow. Gosh, you are exquisitely beautiful when you let go and radiate love.

Be her today.

23 SATURDAY ◑

Haliya reminds you to notice the takay flowers that you created the magic to blossom. They are blooming and weaving magic and beauty throughout your life this weekend.

I wonder what you will see and discover when you look closely.

24 SUNDAY

25 MONDAY

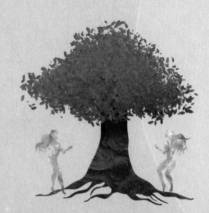

26 TUESDAY

27 WEDNESDAY

28 THURSDAY

With Haliya's help, what can you be extra thankful for today?
We are going to write out three – one about your physical beauty, one about how you shine your light in the world and one about your gifts.

1. With a heart filled with gratitude I am thankful for my _____
because they help me to _____
2. With a heart filled with gratitude I am thankful for the way I _____
because this allows me to _____
3. With a heart filled with gratitude I am thankful for my gift of _____
because this helps me to be amazing at _____

Hands on your heart and take five big, deep breaths filling up your whole body with the gifts that are you this year.

29 FRIDAY

30 SATURDAY

The dark night before the new moon brings you the opportunity to take a last pause before the new moon begins tomorrow. Feeling tired is normal around this time in the moon cycle. Do you have a special need today? What is it? How can you give yourself that to feel an extra dose of support?

1 SUNDAY ○

Today's new moon is the first of two that fall in December. It's the beginning of the black moon cycle, an auspicious time for you! It falls in the fiery sign of Sagittarius and brings in the fire, the passions and the possibilities in your life.

Fire up, baby, this is going to be an exciting month.

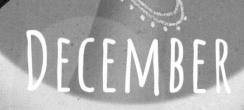

MAYARI

Mayari is a powerhouse Philippine (Tagalog) moon goddess ruler of the night skies, of war, combat, beauty, strength and revolution. Mayari is the most beautiful of all the celestial goddesses from this time, even though she only has one eye.

According to ancient myth, Mayari's father Bathala died without leaving a will. Mayari's brother Apolaki wanted to rule the earth alone, but Mayari wanted to share this task equally. The siblings fought with bamboo clubs until Mayari won, but in the battle, she lost an eye. Discovering what he had done, Apolaki agreed to rule the earth with Mayari – him ruling through the day and her ruling through the night, which is dimmer due to the loss of her eye.

Mayari has come through to support you this month to inspire you to stop striving for perfection in your body, but rather embody all the millions and billions of sacred cells that make up who you are. Each tiny particle comes together to form you. You are divinely beautiful and perfectly imperfect just the way you are.

Mayari's mantra is 'I am learning that physical perfection is a myth, I can choose to love my body exactly as it is today.'

Her crystals are tiger's eye for balance and serpentine for personal strength.

Her totem is the wolf symbolizing the power and strength of the moon and of herself.

Her exercises are combat, weight training and kayaking.

Her scents are dreamy such as frankincense, jasmine, lavender and rose.

2 MONDAY

3 TUESDAY

Sparkle and shine even brighter today, baby. Yeah, and keep smiling like that, it's cute.

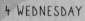

4 WEDNESDAY

5 THURSDAY

6 FRIDAY

7 SATURDAY

When the stress of this time to be perfect comes through, take a breath and say to yourself, 'This year I am choosing ease and joy over stress and angst.' Sway your hips to your goddess self-care toolkit songs and flow with grace through your day.

8 SUNDAY ◑

9 MONDAY

Mayari sends you this message – 'Each cell in your body has been created for you to house the most precious gift: your soul. It is the protector who carries your soul on its journey through this lifetime, to love it in each moment.'

Touch your body all over now. Feel it. Know it. Love it and be thankful for it today.

10 TUESDAY

11 WEDNESDAY

12 THURSDAY

13 FRIDAY

Today is Friday 13th – Day of the Goddess. Tune into your sacred feminine energy today. Wonder at the beauty of you. Nourish your body with moisturizer or spray on an alluring perfume. Light a candle to light up your world with the passion that is you. Flirt with the wind. Drink in the sacred water. Dance through your day on the earth and just radiate your loving medicine everywhere you go.

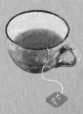

14 SATURDAY

15 SUNDAY ●

Happy full moon, beautiful one. Your last full moon of the year is here and she falls in the airy and dreamy sign of Gemini. Stand under this moon and just bathe in the vitality, the power and the magic of this time. Ask her to settle your mind and shower you in lavish sprinkles of love. Ground in with those big strong tree roots and just breathe it all in, trusting that in the space you have created today, you are in your perfect place.

16 MONDAY

17 TUESDAY

18 WEDNESDAY

19 THURSDAY

It's not always about everyone seeing you sparkle and shine, sometimes the best way to sparkle is to do it for yourself ... and then admire your glow. Singing Christmas carols really loudly, because you can, makes for amazing Christmas glow and sparkly goodness rains through your body ... perhaps you can try that this week?

20 FRIDAY

21 SATURDAY

Winter solstice, a day that begins the new light of the sun's energy: a rebirth. The energy of winter really starts to come through now as nature turns her focus in. Create the space to look at what you want to create during the rest of your year. Just like in nature, you can nurture your dreams now, birthing them into reality in spring.

22 SUNDAY

23 MONDAY

Time to do your new goddess self-care toolkit, using the power and magic of Goddess Mayari. Jump over to your new *Moon Goddess Diary 2025* and let's do this together.

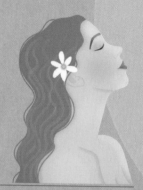

24 TUESDAY

25 WEDNESDAY

What do you love about Christmas? Do that.

How do you want to be treated this year? Give yourself that.

Who do you want to spend it with and for how long? Hang with them!

How can you weave in your Christmas magic, radiant sparkle and exquisite love that little bit more this year, doing and eating and gifting and hugging all those things that fill you up with pleasure? Do that (it so works)!

With a Christmas wink and an extra hug for being oh so special you ... Merry Christmas, baby.

26 THURSDAY

27 FRIDAY

Double new moon month, or a black moon cycle, means that projects and plans you started at the beginning of December may have failed or stalled; it's not over. Don't give up, baby, it's just all processing and conspiring to your greatest advantage. As it always does.

28 SATURDAY

29 SUNDAY

The dark night before each new moon is extra potent as you have a black moon tomorrow.

Breathe into the darkness, allow the leaning in and the awareness to come through. Contemplate.

It's time to get clear by cleansing and releasing any last fragments you have been holding on to and clear any clutter that remains from 2024.

30 MONDAY ○

Happy new moon, darling one. Today, new waves of magical moonbeams spread through your world offering you waves of love and light. She has such a fresh feeling kinda vibe ... can you feel that too?

Your last new moon of 2024 falls in the earthy sign of Capricorn. Stability, direction and grounded movement into your year ahead is what is coming through. She reminds you that anything is possible when you see it, when you feel it, when you believe in your dreams, but most importantly when you take the daily baby steps of action.

I so can't wait to see what you can achieve when you weave that through the whole of your 2025.

31 TUESDAY

Hey beautiful one, I am completely filled with bubbles of love and gratitude that you have chosen to spend your journey through 2024 with me. It is an honor to hold this sacred space for you as you learn to weave in the medicine that is you through your life.

Here's to a magical, expansive and epically light-filled 2025 together ... let's do this!

Nicci x

1 WEDNESDAY

RITUAL TO CLOSE OFF THE YEAR 2024

As you close off the year and begin to walk a new rainbow path into the adventure of 2025, create a little space to do this ritual. Say out loud:

'Today I send gratitude to the path I walked this year, the experiences I had, the people I shared this adventure with. I am so thankful for the learnings I received and the wisdom I called upon from my 12 Moon Goddesses and from inside myself, to support me deeply.

I send thanks to all my angels, my spirits guides, Mother Earth, the seasons, the planets and the moon for holding me as I moved through this year.

I am here today on the last day of this year because I made it through all those tough times, the challenges, the deep ravines of sadness and trauma, the endless mountains of hardship and uncertainty. I kept swimming through the oceans of pain and fear.
I kept moving and walking and pivoting through it all. I chose to keep going – gosh, I'm so proud of me!'

Now put your hands on your hips, broaden your chest, raise your chin and take a big deep breath. Now keep reading aloud!

'I realize now that I am rather amazing! I see that more clearly than I have before.
I am ready to see my magnificence and my potency so much more in 2025. I am ready to use my gifts and talents to value myself and to sprinkle my magic through the world.

My vision will be clear and profound as I follow my dreams, my groove, my light, my way.

In 2025, I am staying open to receiving sprinkles of magic, laughter, joy and hope.

I am ready for my dreams. I am ready for my desires. I am ready to choose me.'

Now happy dance with all the songs you chose to support you this year from your goddess self-care toolkit, swinging into your BEST year yet, you spunky and oh so gorgeous thang!

Grab your 2025 diary now so you can feel extra supported and held while you learn how to accept what is, release the past and allow endings to occur with grace, love and flow.

I'll be there to support you in your transformation.

With radiant sprinkles of love and big smooches.

Nicci xx

There comes a time when you are craving more ...

When you get tired of putting everyone else first, tired of compromising your needs to please those around you and tired of being the peacekeeper.

Where you are ready to learn how to be big, be bold, be seen, be desired and be truly loved.

Where you know that you are wanting to heal so you can feel radiant and free.

Where you want to be reconnected to your inner moon goddess.

Where the whispers of your sacred feminine get louder, stronger and more persistent.

There comes a moment where you can't shut them out any longer, because you know that you are destined for a deeper connection to yourself, your wisdom and your higher levels of support.

I am the expert at this.

I'd be honored to work with you further in my Moon Goddess Academy: www.niccigaraicoa.com/programs/mentoring

With grace and radiant love,

Nicci x

> Nicci Garaicoa is a powerful healer, an intuitive channel of moon goddess and sacred feminine wisdom and the author of five books.
>
> She has a special love for the moon. You can find her daily moon musings and extra sprinkles of love at **f** 📷 @Niccigaraicoa

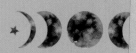

This diary is dedicated
women who nurture the wor
stepmother, co-parent, grand
fur baby and plant moms, the
protectors and caregivers to
For each of you who, despit
obstacles in your way, show u
their darndest to shine your lig
your life.

This edition is f

With radiant beams of light
from my heart to

Nicci x

NB: All moon times and planetary movements used through this diary are set to Greenwich Mean Time (GMT). To convert times to exactly where you are located in the world, I suggest using www.timeanddate.com. Moon and planetary interpretations consider all aspects of where the moon, the sun, the astrological signs and the planets fall on each day and are not taken out of context.

A Rockpool book
PO Box 252
Summer Hill
NSW 2130, Australia

rockpoolpublishing.com
Follow us! **f** 📷 rockpoolpublishing
Tag your images with #rockpoolpublishing

ISBN: 9781922579560, *Northern Hemisphere edition*

Published in 2023 by Rockpool Publishing
Design by Sara Lindberg, Rockpool Publishing
Edited by Brooke Halliwell

Copyright text © Nicci Garaicoa, 2023
Copyright illustrations © Olivia Bürki, 2023
Copyright design © Rockpool Publishing, 2023

Printed and bound in China
10 9 8 7 6 5 4 3 2 1